An Introduction to Dermatological Surgery

An Introduction to Dermatological Surgery

CLIFFORD LAWRENCE
Consultant Dermatologist
Royal Victoria Infirmary
Newcastle Upon Tyne

WITH A CONTRIBUTION FROM
GERARD PANTING
Head of UK Medical Services
The Medical Protection Society
Leeds

Sponsored by

 UCB Pharma

**Blackwell
Science**

© 1996 by
Blackwell Science Ltd
Editorial Offices:
Osney Mead, Oxford OX2 0EL
25 John Street, London WC1N 2BL
23 Ainslie Place, Edinburgh EH3 6AJ
238 Main Street, Cambridge
    Massachusetts 02142, USA
54 University Street, Carlton
    Victoria 3053, Australia

Other Editorial Offices:
Arnette Blackwell SA
    224, Boulevard Saint Germain
    75007 Paris, France

Blackwell Wissenschafts-Verlag GmbH
    Kurfürstendamm 57
    10707 Berlin, Germany

    Zehetnergasse 6
    A-1140 Wien
    Austria

First published 1996

Set by Semantic Graphics, Singapore
Printed and bound in Italy
by G. Canale & C. SpA, Turin

The Blackwell Science logo is a
trade mark of Blackwell Science Ltd,
registered at the United Kingdom
Trade Marks Registry

DISTRIBUTORS

Marston Book Services Ltd
PO Box 269
Abingdon
Oxon OX14 4YN
(*Orders:* Tel: 01235 465500
            Fax: 01235 465555)

USA
Blackwell Science, Inc.
238 Main Street
Cambridge, MA 02142
(*Orders:* Tel: 800 215-1000
            617 876-7000
            Fax: 617 492-5263)

Canada
Copp Clark, Ltd
2775 Matheson Blvd East
Mississauga, Ontario
Canada, L4W 4P7
(*Orders:* Tel: 800 263-4374
            905 238-6074)

Australia
Blackwell Science Pty Ltd
54 University Street
Carlton, Victoria 3053
(*Orders:* Tel: 3 9347 0300
            Fax: 3 9347 5001)

A catalogue record for this title
is available from the British Library

ISBN 0-86542-964-2

Library of Congress
Cataloging-in-publication Data

Lawrence, Clifford M.
    An introduction to
        dermatological surgery /
        Clifford Lawrence, Gerard Panting
        p.   cm.
    Includes bibliographical references
    and index.
    ISBN 0-86542-964-2
    1. Skin—surgery.
    I. Panting, Gerard.   II. Title.
    [DNLM: 1. Skin—surgery.
    2. Surgery, Operative—methods.
    WR 100L419i   1996]
    RD520.L39   1996
    617.4′77—dc20
    DNLM/DLC
    for Library of Congress   96-8184
                                             CIP

Contents

Preface

This book attempts to describe the principles, limitations and indications of techniques used in basic dermatological surgery in sufficient detail to enable the reader to attempt the simpler procedures, after a brief period of supervised training. I have assumed that the reader is able to make a confident clinical diagnosis but has very little pre-existing knowledge of dermatological surgical techniques. The book is aimed at general practitioners performing skin surgery. Dermatologists in training should be familiar with all the techniques described, but will require additional reading to cover the subject completely. It is anticipated that non-specialists performing these techniques will recognize the need for additional training in dermatological diagnosis—the key to efficient and effective skin surgery.

Acknowledgements

Writing a book is like climbing one of Wainwright's dome-shaped lakeland mountains. You keep thinking you are near the top only to find that there is still a little further to go. I survived this climb with the encouragement, patience and good humour of my wife Anne and children Tom, Jo, Chris and James who have quietly endured evenings and weekends with Dad 'tapping away on the 'puter'. Steve Pedler, Phil Adams, Margaret Johnson, Bruce Burnett and Rod Bexton all provided much appreciated expert advice. I am very grateful to Gerard Panting who has kindly provided an expert's view on the medico-legal aspects of skin surgery. Several of the chapters cover topics included at the British Society of Dermatological Surgery Annual Workshop, where I have had the privilege to lecture and demonstrate since their creation in 1984. I have consciously or otherwise adopted ideas and advice given by other speakers at these meetings and I acknowledge their contribution. Neil Cox took the time to read the manuscript and made lots of typically useful and salient suggestions, but any remaining mistakes are mine.

1: Introduction

Introduction

The appealing quality of skin surgery is its simplicity and effectiveness. This simplicity is, however, not a justification for surgery without adequate indication. It is a mistake to assume that an elliptical excision or biopsy is required when faced with an undiagnosed rash or skin lump. Diagnosis must come before surgery. Without an accurate differential diagnosis, surgery may be performed unnecessarily, a potentially more scarring technique chosen or a tumour incompletely excised. A range of techniques can be used for many common benign skin disorders (Table 1.1), although one very simple method may produce optimal results. When cryotherapy is used the clinical diagnosis must be accurate as no histological confirmation is obtained. Furthermore, because cryotherapy is easily done incorrectly, some lesions frozen by enthusiasts are best not treated by the non-specialist (Chapter 17). This book will emphasize this principle and illustrate the basic techniques used in dermatological surgery. Before undertaking any procedure the points listed in Table 1.2 should be considered.

Is surgery necessary?

Not all lumps have to be removed. Reassurance is frequently sufficient for benign lesions. Alternative treatments, including cryotherapy or radiotherapy, may produce superior results. Do not assume that because a lump exists and a diagnosis cannot be made, it must be excised. A second opinion from a specialist may be more appropriate.

Choose the correct surgical procedure

The correct surgical procedure depends critically on the differential diagnosis. Without this you are unable to decide if surgery is necessary, the type and extent of treatment, or guide the pathologist in interpreting the specimen.

Do not over-reach yourself

Avoid attempting a procedure unless you are completely familiar with it.

Be aware of the potential cosmetic results

Make sure the patient understands that surgery inevitably means that a scar will be left. This scar may be barely noticeable or potentially disfiguring. It is usually possible to reassure the patient that the final result will be better than the existing defect; if this is not probable, let the patient know what the final cosmetic result will look like. It is easier to defend extensive or potentially scarring surgery when treating a malignancy. By contrast, if a benign lesion is unnecessarily or inappropriately treated, it may be more difficult to justify a poor cosmetic result. Excision of a benign lesion on a keloid-prone site or individual should be avoided (see Fig. 7.3).

Malignancies

When treating malignant tumours, always treat the excision and closure as two separate operations. Never compromise the adequacy of the excision to make the closure easier; recurrences are more difficult to treat than primary tumours.

Table 1.1 Management of common benign lesions.

Lesion and symptom	Cryotherapy	Curette	Shave	Excision	Other	Reassure
Naevus, pale, cosmetic	X	X	✔	✔	X	✔
Naevus, protuberant, benign, catches on clothing etc.	X	X	✔	X	X	X
Naevus, itchy, benign	X	X	✔ May fail if itch is due to follicular irritation	✔	X	✔
Naevus, deeply pigmented or hairy	X	X	✔ Hairs and pigment may remain	✔	X	If no clinical suspicion
Naevus, suspicious	X	X	X	✔	X	X
Dermatofibroma, itchy	Specialist only	X	X	✔	Intralesional steroids (specialist only)	✔
Dermatofibroma, cosmetic	X	X	X	May leave poor scar	X	✔
Seborrhoeic keratosis	✔	✔	X	Only if diagnosis uncertain	X	✔
Haemangioma	✔	X	X	✔	Laser therapy	✔
Chondrodermatitis nodularis	Specialist only	X	X	Cartilage excision	Intralesional or topical steroids	X
Pyogenic granuloma	Specialist only	✔	X	✔	X	X
Viral wart	✔	✔	X	X	See Chapter 16	✔
Skin tag	✔	X	✔	✔ If very large	Electrodesiccate small tags	✔
Epidermoid cyst	X	X	X	✔	Decompression and excision (Chapter 14)	✔
Lipoma	X	X	X	✔	Liposuction	✔
Spider naevus	✔	X	X	X	Laser therapy Cold-point cautery Electrodesiccate	✔ Especially children

Biopsy of skin tumours or unknown lumps, prior to referral to a specialist

This is commonly a waste of time and resources. A pretreatment biopsy is only justified when there is doubt about the clinical diagnosis or the patient is being referred directly to a radiotherapist. In most instances confirmation of the clinical diagnosis is obtained as part of the curative procedure.

Table 1.2 A pre-excision differential diagnosis is important for the following reasons.

Benign lesions do not need to be excised
If the surgery is unnecessary and the cosmetic results are poor, the patient may be dissatisfied
Elliptical excision may not be the treatment of choice. Other surgical therapies may give better cosmetic results
The recommended margin of normal skin that should be excised around a tumour depends on the type of tumour
The patient needs to be aware of the potential diagnosis before surgery

Biopsy of rashes

The skin has a limited range of histological responses. Correct interpretation of these changes depends critically on the operator choosing the correct biopsy site, obtaining an adequate specimen and providing an accurate differential diagnosis so that the pathologist is able to interpret the biopsy appearances correctly.

Specimens

Send all specimens for histological inspection (Chapter 21) as this provides confirmation of the clinical diagnosis and will ultimately improve diagnostic accuracy. Failure to do so may result in an important missed diagnosis.

Biopsy book

Keep a record of all procedures in a biopsy book with the clinical diagnosis so that the histology result can be compared with the clinical diagnosis and results are not overlooked.

Follow up your patients

Much can be learnt by following up patients you have operated on. Whilst gaining expertise in a technique, review patients frequently to observe the changes. This will familiarize you with the expected wound appearance in the first few weeks. Cosmetic results continue to improve for up to a year after most skin surgery. After treating a malignancy, follow up the patient for an appropriate period to exclude a recurrence or new tumour formation (Chapter 18).

Further reading

Champion RH, Burton JL & Ebling FJG (eds) (1992) *Textbook of Dermatology*, 5th edn. Blackwell Scientific Publications, Oxford.
Habif TR (1990) *Clinical Dermatology: A Color Guide to Diagnosis and Therapy*, 2nd edn. Mosby, St Louis.
Lawrence CM (1991) The treatment of chondrodermatitis nodularis with cartilage removal alone. *Arch Dermatol.* **127**: 530–535.
Jackson A (1995) Prevention, early detection and team management of skin cancer in primary care: contribution to The Health of the Nation objectives. *Br J Gen Pract* **45**: 97–101.
Lawrence CM & Cox NH (1993) *Physical Signs in Dermatology. A Color Atlas and Text.* Mosby–Wolfe, London.
MacKie RM (1989) *Skin Cancer*. Martin Dunitz, London.

2: Equipment

Many skin surgical techniques are essentially simple, rapid procedures that only require a clinically clean environment and simple equipment. It is none the less important to perform these and more complex operations in the best possible circumstances and before considering the instruments required it is essential to obtain suitable operating facilities.

Operating facilities

Room

A dedicated clinically clean procedure room, approximately 3.5 × 3.5 metres (12 × 12 ft) in size, close enough to other clinical areas for assistance to be obtained if required, should be used. Uncluttered, easily cleaned work surfaces and storage space for instruments and suture material should be available. A mobile stainless-steel trolley for holding instruments is essential.

Table

A static examination couch and a wall-mounted light are just adequate for curettage and shave excision. This arrangement, however, will reduce your ability to provide optimum results as it will not always be possible to position yourself optimally to reach the affected area. Furthermore, using a fixed couch will exhaust the operator by causing him/her to stoop. An operating table or couch that can be raised to the appropriate height is essential if lengthy procedures are attempted. An electrically operated dentist's chair is suitable for lesions on the head and neck, but not those on the trunk and limbs. The table should be placed in the middle of the room so that there is access from all sides. The foot of the table must be able to be tilted upwards so that

patient's feet can be elevated if he/she faints while lying flat.

Lamp

A ceiling-mounted, swivelling and hinged lamp with more than one bulb is ideal. Such a lamp usually requires a specially built ceiling mounting and this will add to the expense. In most rooms with wooden ceiling joists only a single-bulb, hinged light can be fitted. Floor-based lights are cumbersome and occupy a lot of valuable floor space (Fig. 2.1).

Safety features and resuscitation equipment

The table must be sited so that the operator can get behind the patient to insert an airway if required and it must be possible to tip the table so

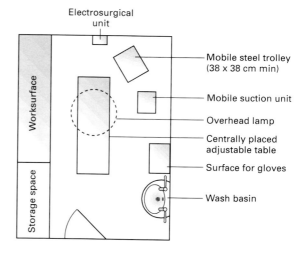

Fig. 2.1 Plan of suitable surgery room. A 3.5 metre (12 ft) square room is an appropriate size. The table should be in the centre of the room so that the patient can be reached from any side. A ceiling-mounted operating light is necessary.

Table 2.1 Possible emergency equipment and apparatus.

Equipment
Tipping table with access behind the patient's head
Portable artificial ventilation, e.g. Ambu bag
Airways
Portable suction apparatus
Oxygen supply
Disposable needles, syringes, intravenous cannulae
Intravenous fluids

Emergency drugs
Chlorpheniramine maleate 5 × 1 ml ampoules (10-mg/vial)
Hydrocortisone sodium succinate 5 × 100 mg for injection
Adrenaline 0.5 ml 1/1000 5 ampoules
Diazepam 5 × 2 ml

Note: This list is neither exhaustive nor mandatory. Individuals must decide what equipment is appropriate to their practice.

that it can be placed head-down if the patient faints. Ideally, the room exit should be wide enough to allow access with a trolley. Suggested resuscitation equipment is listed (Table 2.1). There are no legal requirements and the range of equipment carried will depend on the operator's judgement, based on the nature and extent of the surgery performed.

Sterile procedures and equipment

A sterile sheet covering that part of the patient immediately adjacent to the operation site is useful to rest instruments on and to prevent contamination of sutures. The simplest is a towel with a 7.5 cm (3 in) hole in the centre which can be draped over the patient, with the wound exposed through the hole. Patients may not like being covered by the towel and sometimes two towels laid either side of the lesion with the patient's nose and mouth exposed are preferred. If paper sheets are used, these must be water-resistant or they will cease to be a sterile screen once wet.

Operating assistants

Always try to operate with an assistant to supply suture material, cut sutures, reassure the patient, provide missing pieces of equipment and, if necessary, run for assistance. A gloved operating assistant to hold suction equipment and retract skin edges is also useful during complex procedures.

Suction

Suction is not essential but during excision surgery suction makes operating easier and faster. An assistant must be available to hold and direct the suction tip. A small electrically operated mobile suction machine can be used for operation suction and as part of the resuscitation equipment. Listen to the noise level before purchasing the machine as a noisy machine can be a nuisance.

Diathermy (high-frequency electrosurgery) equipment

An electrosurgical unit can be used for intraoperative haemostasis and any procedure where electrocautery might be used (Chapter 5).

Skin preparation

No skin preparation is ideal and none will completely sterilize the skin. Do not use alcohol-based solutions because of the fire risk with cautery and electrosurgery. Aqueous chlorhexidine solution or povidone-iodine is probably most commonly used. Sponge cubes or gauze swabs should be held in sponge holders before being dipped into the sterilizing solution and rubbed on the skin.

Hand-washing

Hand-washing must be done properly to avoid the risk of cross-infection if a glove is damaged or faulty (Fig. 2.2). Elbow-action taps are needed.

Gloves and protective clothing

Wear gloves for all procedures for your own protection. Disposable non-sterile gloves are quite

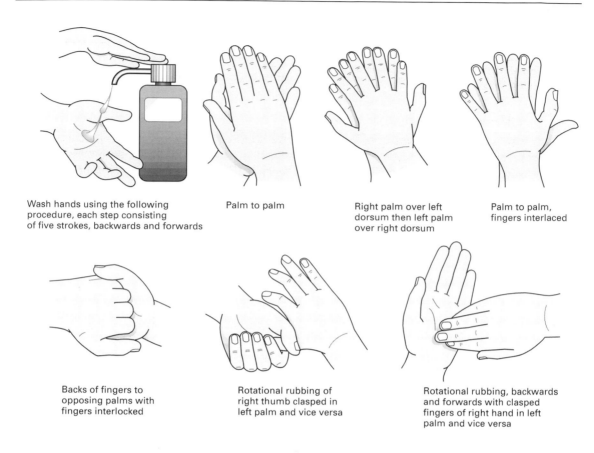

Wash hands using the following procedure, each step consisting of five strokes, backwards and forwards

Palm to palm

Right palm over left dorsum then left palm over right dorsum

Palm to palm, fingers interlaced

Backs of fingers to opposing palms with fingers interlocked

Rotational rubbing of right thumb clasped in left palm and vice versa

Rotational rubbing, backwards and forwards with clasped fingers of right hand in left palm and vice versa

Fig. 2.2 Hand-washing technique. (From Field EA, Jedynakiewicz NM & King CM (1992) A practical gloving and handwashing regimen for dental practice. *Br Dent J* **172**: 111–113, with permission.)

adequate for curettage and shave biopsies. Sterile gloves should be used for suture surgery. A disposable pinafore or gown is useful to protect clothing. Masks and eye shields are not essential but do protect against the risk of blood splashes.

Skin shaving

If required, skin should be shaved immediately before surgery and not in the preceding 24 hours as this damages the skin surface and greatly increases staphylococcal carriage and hence the risk of secondary infection. Clipping the hair rather than shaving is usually just as effective, does not damage the skin surface and has the advantage that the direction of the hair shaft is preserved and hence any incision can be made parallel to and not through the hair follicle (see page 57).

Operating instruments

It is convenient to use a selection of instruments in a pack which contains sterile towels and chambers or a gallipot for skin preparation solution; these may be obtained from a local hospital. For some procedures it is more economical to use individually packed instruments. Inexpensive surgical equipment tends to be poorly made, wears out easily and is usually too heavy, clumsy or large for optimum results. The plastic surgery and ophthalmology sections of manufacturers' brochures contain the type of equipment used in skin surgery. Equipment should be reasonably delicate, easy to handle and an appropriate size (Table 2.2).

Table 2.2 Surgical equipment.

	Desirable features	Undesirable features	Suggested type
Scalpel handle and blade	Disposable versions are excellent No. 15 blade is the most appropriate for skin surgery The round Beaver handle may be preferred	Larger handle, e.g. no. 4 or larger blade, is unnecessary	No. 3 Bard-Parker handle with no. 15 blade Beaver (pencil-shaped) handle
Needle-holders	Small, light-weight needle-holders. Ensure the hinge joint does not snag the suture material as the knot is thrown. Choose smooth or very finely serrated jaws. These will not damage fine suture material	Wide jaws flatten out fine curved needles Coarsely serrated jaws damage suture material or the suture slips between the serrations	Halsey, box needle-holder Webster needle-holder Nievert needle-holder
Non-toothed forceps	The ends must meet properly	Pointed forceps are not useful for routine work. Heavy forceps with large tips are not appropriate. The handles must spring back into shape properly	Adson non-toothed forceps
Tooth forceps	2 : 1 teeth with fine tips	Very large teeth will crush tissue Cheaper versions are made from softer metal and easily become misshapen	Adson tooth forceps
Small straight scissors	Straight/sharp 4½-in scissors — do not use these for cutting sutures or dressings if you also intend to use them for cutting tissue	Large or blunt scissors are not appropriate	Iris scissors
Suture and dressing scissors	Blunt or rounded ends avoid the risk of a trembling assistant injuring the patient	Do not use fine or quality scissors for cutting sutures. This will blunt them very quickly	Standard sharp/blunt blunt/blunt straight 5-in
Skin hook	7–8-in long single hook with an oblong cross-sectional handle so that hook direction is always obvious and the instrument does not roll away	Hook size has to be correct, i.e. approximately 3 mm in diameter. Smaller hooks are not usually robust enough and larger hooks are too big for skin surgery	Gillies large
Artery forceps	Fine small end 4–5 in long. Curved ends are easier to use than straight forceps		Halsted mosquito box artery forceps
Suture removal forceps	Flat ends approximately 4–5 in long Depilatory forceps are the best	Fine-tipped forceps are no use. They usually do not meet at the end and the suture material cannot be grasped easily Plastic forceps are designed for a non-touch dressing technique, not for suture removal. Suture removal blades are not satisfactory (see Chapter 6)	Whitfield's depilatory forceps
Curved scissors	Flat, blunt points 4–5 in long. Serrated blades greatly improve cutting quality	Large or bulky curved scissors are not appropriate. Pointed-end curved scissors should not be used for undermining	Kilner scissors Metzenbaum scissors

Skin marking

Bonney's blue or specially designed skin marker operating pens should be used to mark the skin and not ballpoint or felt-tipped pens as these contain pigments that potentially may permanently tattoo the skin. Bonney's blue can be tattooed into the skin with the tip of the pen nib to create a mark that will resist washing off but fade completely after 3–4 days. A Sommerlad pen is expensive but the best sterilizable pen available.

Practice points

• The jaws of more expensive needle-holders, forceps and scissors are sometimes faced with specially hardened tungsten-carbide tips to increase the strength and stability of the grip on the needle or, in the case of scissors, to prolong the life of the cutting edge.
• Gold-plated handles on some expensive pieces of equipment help distinguish them as delicate items that should be handled carefully.
• Skin hooks can be used as an alternative to toothed forceps, which tend to crush tissue if used too heavily. Skin hooks are dangerous and, of all the instruments used, the one most likely to injure the surgeon or nurse. Skin hooks should not be used when operating on a high-risk patient.
• Grasp the needle-holder, correcting with the index finger on the jaws near the needle, the thumb half-way down and the handle held in the palm. Do not place the fingers in the rings. Using this palm grip it is easier to rotate the needle-holder when using a curved needle and finer fingertip control is achieved. It is also possible, with practice, to open the jaws by pushing forward with the base of the thumb.

Further reading

Bennett RC (1988) Chapter 7 Instruments and their care. In: *Fundamentals of Cutaneous Surgery*. CV Mosby, St Louis.

Cawson RA, Curson I & Whittington DR (1983) The hazards of dental local anaesthetics. *Br Dent J* **154**: 253–258.

Fewkes JL, Cheney ML & Pollack SV (1992) *Illustrated Atlas of Cutaneous Surgery*. JB Lippincott, Philadelphia.

Grande DJ & Neuberg M (1989) Instrumentation for the dermatologic surgeon. *J Dermatol Surg Oncol* **15**: 288–297.

Perks ER (1977) The diagnosis and management of sudden collapse in dental practice. *Br Dent J* **143**: 307–310.

3: Sterilization of surgical equipment

Equipment sterilized professionally and delivered to the surgery is a convenient and satisfactory method. When steam or gas sterilization techniques are used, packed sterile instruments would normally be given a shelf-life of around 12 months. Single-use disposable instruments, dressing materials and sutures are also very useful. If surgical equipment has to be sterilized in the surgery, the only practical and acceptable method is a small portable autoclave. Other methods are less satisfactory or ineffective (Table 3.1). Before sterilization all instruments must be cleaned to remove tissue or blood by scrubbing with soap and water. Specialized ultrasound cleaning equipment can also be used but is expensive and unnecessary for the robust instruments used in skin surgery.

Types of sterilization

Boiling water

Boiling water does not destroy all bacterial spores. Hepatitis virus is destroyed by boiling for approximately 10 minutes.

Cold sterilization (chemical sterilization)

Glutaraldehyde is widely used for the sterilization of flexible scopes. Immersion times of 3 hours are required for spore-bearing organisms and 1 hour for mycobacteria. The 4-minute immersion time used in some gastroscopy units is only long enough to destroy *Helicobacter pylori*, hepatitis virus and human immunodeficiency virus (HIV). A gastroscope treated in this way can be considered to be disinfected but not sterilized. More importantly, glutaraldehyde is a potential hazard to staff as it causes respiratory and skin irritation and sensitization. The rules governing

Table 3.1 Comparison of sterilization techniques.

Technique	Time required to kill bacteria, fungi, viruses and spores	Comments
Boiling water	30 minutes Bacterial spores not killed	Do not use
Glutaraldehyde (Cidex)	15 minutes Mycobacteria 60 minutes Spores 3 hours	Tarnishes steel instruments Dangerous chemical, skin and lung irritant and sensitizer
Dry heat	1–2 hours at 160°C	Too slow; may warp metal objects
Autoclave	15–20 minutes Scrapie prion (Creutzfeldt–Jakob disease) requires sodium hypochlorite cleaning followed by autoclaving for 60 minutes	Quick, effective Dulls sharp instruments
Gas	1–8 hours	Dangerous chemical Not suitable for bench-top system

the safe handling of this material mean that it should no longer be used without taking expensive precautions. It is thus not an option for the sterilization of surgical equipment.

Dry heat sterilization

Dry heat is a less efficient sterilizing medium than wet heat because bacterial spores are much more resistant to dry heat, possibly because spores are naturally water-free and have evolved in this way to survive temperature extremes. Hence, higher temperatures and longer times are required to achieve similar results. A hot-air oven with an uninterrupted cycle which includes a holding time of 60 minutes at 160°C can be effective but when the warm-up and cool-down time is added, the total cycle time is very long. Furthermore, in the USA a 2-hour holding time at 160°C is recommended. Few currently available hot-air ovens have the required timed cycle with an automatic door-locking device.

Autoclave

Steam sterilization is fast and reliable. Most steam autoclaves operate at 121°C (pressure 100 kPa) with a holding time of 15 minutes. Raising the temperature to 126–129°C reduces the time to 10 minutes and a temperature of 134–138°C requires a holding time of 3 minutes (cycle time 15–20 minutes). The holding time refers to the time during which the specified temperature is maintained. The total cycle time will always be longer, as this includes the warm-up, cool-down and drying times. Instruments must be cleaned and dried, and hinged instruments should be opened before sterilization so that the steam gets to all surfaces. The method has the disadvantage of dulling sharp steel, and instruments may rust if not left to dry adequately. Once sterile, instruments must be used and cannot be stored in holding solutions.

The sterilization of packed instruments in portable autoclaves is not recommended by the Department of Health. In a portable steam steril-izer air is displaced by the hot steam entering the sterilizing chamber, unlike a hospital-style autoclave where the air is pumped out. It is thus possible for air to remain in the sterilizer or in a porous load, which will prevent satisfactory sterilization. Furthermore, since there is no vacuum-drying stage, most loads are still wet at the end of the cycle and are thus not suitable for storage. This inability to sterilize packed instruments is a problem for all manufacturers as a sterilizer that incorporates the type of vacuum pump required by the British Standard becomes too big to be portable and much more expensive.

Gas sterilization

Ethylene oxide sterilization is used for materials that would be damaged by the temperatures used in an autoclave. The equipment required is large and expensive and the ethylene oxide used is potentially hazardous. There is no bench-top apparatus commercially available in the UK.

Further reading

Cowan RE, Manning AP, Aycliffe GAJ *et al.* (1993) Aldehyde disinfectants and health in endoscopy units. *Gut* **34**: 1641–1645.

Department of Health (1990) *A Further Evaluation of Transportable Steam Sterilisers for Unwrapped Instruments and Utensils* (ref. HEI no. 196). Available from DHSS NHS Procurement Directorate, Room 423, 14 Russell Square, London WC1B 5EP Tel 0171 972 8189.

Sebben JE (1984) Sterilization and care of surgical instruments and supplies. *J Am Acad Dermatol* **11**: 381–392.

Sebben JE (1988) Survey of sterile technique used by dermatologic surgeons. *J Am Acad Dermatol* **18**: 1107–1113.

4: Local anaesthetics

Type of anaesthetic

Several types of local anaesthetic are available with slightly different durations of anaesthetic effect and potential toxicity. Lignocaine (lidocaine) is widely available, inexpensive and rarely causes allergic reactions. The duration of effect of lignocaine with adrenaline is similar to the longer-acting local anaesthetics (plain bupivacaine and etidocaine). These advantages of lignocaine make it the drug of choice for skin surgery and only one other alternative agent is briefly described.

Lignocaine and lignocaine with adrenaline injection constituents

Pain lignocaine is simply a mixture of lignocaine and water. Adding adrenaline causes local vasoconstriction and hence reduced anaesthetic clearance. This results in a prolonged local effect (Table 4.1) and reduced risk of systemic toxicity,

Table 4.1 Duration of effect of lignocaine anaesthetics after infiltration anaesthesia.

Anaesthetic	Available as	Maximum safe adult dose* (limiting ingredient)	Approximate duration of anaesthesia (hours)
0.5% lignocaine plain	10 ml ampoule 20 ml multidose vial	40 ml (contains 200 mg lignocaine)	1 ½
0.5% lignocaine plus 1 : 200 00 adrenaline	20 ml multidose vial	40 ml (contains 200 mg lignocaine and 200 µg adrenaline	4
1% lignocaine plain	2–20 ml ampoules 20 ml multidose vial	20 ml (contains 200 mg lignocaine)	2
1% lignocaine plus 1 : 200 000 adrenaline	20 ml multidose vial	40 ml (Contains 400 mg lignocaine and 200 µg adrenaline)	7
2% lignocaine plain	2–5 ml ampoules 20 ml multidose vial	10 ml (contains 200 mg lignocaine)	2
2% lignocaine plus 1 : 200 000 adrenaline	20 ml multidose vial	25 ml (contains 500 mg lignocaine and 125 µg adrenaline)	5–7
2% lignocaine plus 1 : 80 000 adrenaline	1.8 ml dental cartridges	16 ml (contains 320 mg lignocaine and 200 µg adrenaline)	No data†

*Assumes an adult can tolerate 500 mg of lignocaine when mixed with adrenaline, 200 mg lignocaine when used without adrenaline and 200 µg adrenaline. Use half this amount in patients at risk from lignocaine toxicity (Table 4.4).
†1 : 80 000 and 1 : 200 000 adrenaline with lignocaine produce the same duration of nerve block anaesthesia. There appears to be little objective rationale for the use of 1 : 80 000 adrenaline in dental anaesthetic solutions.
Note: The amount of vasoconstrictor in the solution has historically been expressed as a dilution, whereas the amount of anaesthetic is expressed as a concentration (e.g. a 1 : 200 000 *dilution* represents a *concentration* of 1 g in 200 000 ml of solution i.e. 1000/200 000 mg/ml = 0.005 mg/ml = 5 µg/ml; similarly 1 : 1000 = 1 mg/ml = 1000 µg/ml).

11

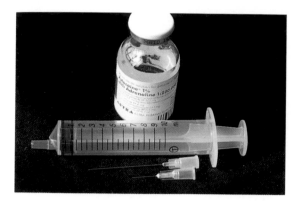

Fig. 4.1 Local anaesthetic. 1% lignocaine plus 1 : 200 000 adrenaline provides optimal duration of anaesthesia and vasoconstriction for skin infiltration anaesthesia. Higher concentrations of either component add little greater benefit. Long thin 27-gauge or short 30-gauge needles are available.

hence more can be injected compared to plain lignocaine. An important added benefit to the skin surgeon is that vasoconstriction results in a relatively blood free operating field. Adrenaline 1 : 200 000 (5 µg/ml) produces optimal skin vasoconstriction and 1% lignocaine plus adrenaline results in a maximal duration of effect (Table 4.1). This combination is equally effective for infiltration anaesthesia and simple nerve blocks and is thus optimal for skin surgery (Fig. 4.1). Increasing the adrenaline concentration to 1 : 80 000 adds no greater anaesthetic duration or vasoconstriction advantage.

Sodium metabisulphite or bisulphite are used when adrenaline is added to prevent adrenaline oxidation (Table 4.2). These chemicals also increase the acidity of the mixture and make the injection more painful. Other factors that contribute to the pain of injections and measures to reduce this effect are listed in Table 4.3. Parabens (syn. hydroxybenzoates, E214-219, and especially methyl and butyl-4-hydroxybenzoate) are added to multi-dose lignocaine vials, but not

Table 4.2 Other ingredients in lignocaine local anaesthetics.

Multi-dose vials	Parabens (hydroxybenzoates)
Anaesthetics with added adrenaline	Sodium bisulphite or metabisulphite

Table 4.3 Suggested methods of making local anaesthetic injections less painful.

Patient preparation
Relaxed but prepared
Topical EMLA

Equipment
Use long thin (27-gauge) needles

Adapting the anaesthetic
Warm the local anaesthetic
Use plain lignocaine
If adrenaline-containing lignocaine is used, neutralize the
  acidity by mixing with sodium bicarbonate before injection

Injection technique
Manipulate the adjacent skin to distract
Introduce needle gently — do not jab!
Inject slowly
Inject into subcutaneous tissue rather than dermis
Inject into a follicle opening

Delivery
Use nerve blocks if possible and give these through the
  mucosa when possible
Make the first injection as close as possible to the
  innervating nerve

EMLA, eutectic mixture of local anaesthetic.

dental vials. This group of preservatives are recognized allergens widely used in creams and cosmetics. Allergic reactions to anaesthetics are sometimes due to one of these added ingredients rather than the anaesthetic.

Local anaesthetics achieve their effect after diffusion through the myelin sheath around the nerve. Larger fibres have a thicker myelin sheath. Thus, the smaller sensory fibres carrying pain and temperature are more readily blocked than larger fibres carrying touch, vibration, pressure and motor function. Pressure sensation may thus still be present when pain sensation is lost. More importantly temporary local anaesthetic induced motor nerve paralysis can appear during surgery.

Potential side-effects

Lignocaine side-effects

Lignocaine is metabolized in the liver and after

Table 4.4 Patients at greater risk of developing potentially toxic lignocaine blood levels.

Physiological
Elderly
Children

Pathological
Heart failure
Renal failure
Chronic liver disease

Drug interactions
Concurrent administration of cimetidine, β-blockers,
    amiodarone, disopyramide

Table 4.5 Toxicity symptoms of lignocaine.

Low blood levels: 1–5 μg/ml
Increased anxiety
Talkativeness
Tinnitus
Tingling and numbness of the lips and tongue
Nausea and vomiting
Metallic taste
Double vision

Moderate levels: 5–8 μg/ml
Nystagmus
Muscle twitching
Tremor

High levels: 8–12 μg/ml
Convulsions
Respiratory arrest

biliary recycling is excreted in the kidneys. Lignocaine excretion is reduced in the elderly, children and patients with liver, renal or cardiac failure (Table 4.4). Lignocaine is excreted in breast milk but the levels produced are very low and of no toxicological significance. Nursing mothers can continue to breast feed. In a healthy individual large volumes of lignocaine can be given before toxic levels are reached (Table 4.5). In a very extensive procedure, such as a scalp reduction, levels (i.e. 0.6–3.3 μg/ml) similar to that reached when lignocaine is used to treat cardiac arrhythmias (i.e. therapeutic range 1–10 μg/ml) may be achieved after infiltration of 20–50 ml of 2% lignocaine with adrenaline. Perhaps more commonly, accidental intravascular injection may produce transient toxic blood levels. Early side-effects include lightheadedness, anxiety, metallic taste and tinnitus.

Adrenaline side-effects

The vasoconstriction produced by adrenaline increases the amount of anaesthetic that can be injected (Table 4.1), by slowing clearance from the injection site, and reduces bleeding. However, adrenaline may precipitate an arrhythmia or angina in patients with ischaemic heart disease. The addition of adrenaline increases the range of potential drug interactions (Table 4.6) with the local anaesthetic and makes the injection more painful. It is important to remember that whilst the analgesic effect takes approximately 5 minutes to develop, optimal vasoconstriction takes 10–15 minutes.

Prolonged vasoconstriction is the most important side effect of adrenaline. Only plain lignocaine should be used on the fingers, toes and penis. Lignocaine plus adrenaline can be used on the nose and ears, although judgement should be used in diabetic patients with small vessel disease who may have impaired peripheral perfusion. Accidental intravascular injection of anaesthetic containing adrenaline may produce distressing transient side-effects, including tachycardia, anxiety, tremor and hypertension in a healthy individual.

Contraindications to the use of adrenaline

These relate mainly to the potential for producing arrhythmias or angina in predisposed subjects (Table 4.7) and the risk of hypertension in patients with phaeochromocytoma or *uncontrolled* hyperthyroidism.

Local anaesthetics in pregnancy

Fears about the safety of adrenaline in pregnancy were raised when it was demonstrated in experimental animals that adrenaline reduces uterine blood flow. No correlating problem has been

Table 4.6 Potential drug interactions with lignocaine local anaesthetics.

Drug	Effect	Comment
Interactions with lignocaine Amiodarone β-blockers Disopyramide Cimetidine (not ranitidine)	Tend to increase lignocaine levels (various mechanisms)	Concurrent administration of these drugs is not a contraindication to the use of plain lignocaine for anaesthesia. Smaller maximum doses of lignocaine are appropriate in patients taking these drugs who also have other risk factors for lignocaine toxicity (Table 4.4)
Interactions with adrenaline Tricyclic antidepressants, e.g. imipramine, amitriptyline, clomipramine, dothiepin, nortriptyline, trimipramine	Hypertension and tachycardia Ventricular arrhythmias	Use plain lignocaine. Avoid adrenaline-containing local anaesthetics, although it is unlikely that the small quantities of adrenaline contained in < 5 ml of local anaesthetic will result in an adverse reaction. For more prolonged anaesthesia, use prilocaine with felypressin or plain bupivacaine
Non-selective β-blockers, e.g. propranolol, oxprenolol, pindolol, timolol	Hypertension and bradycardia	Avoid adrenaline-containing local anaesthetics. Use plain lignocaine or bupivacaine. Adrenaline can be used in patients taking selective β-blockers (e.g. acebutolol, atenolol, metoprolol)

demonstrated in humans and the conclusion of obstetric anaesthetists is that adrenaline can be used in mid to late pregnancy. Although there is no evidence that small doses of lignocaine and adrenaline given early in pregnancy may harm the fetus, it is probably prudent to delay non-urgent procedures until after the first trimester.

Table 4.7 Situations where adrenaline-containing anaesthetics should be avoided.

Allergy
Demonstrated allergy to sodium metabisulphite

Severe heart disease
Unstable angina, i.e. severe angina unresponsive to medical therapy
Myocardial infarction in previous 6 months
Coronary artery bypass surgery in last 3 months
Refractory ventricular arrhythmias
Untreated or uncontrolled hypertension
Untreated or uncontrolled cardiac failure

Severe endocrine disease
Uncontrolled hyperthyroidism
Uncontrolled diabetes
Phaeochromocytoma

Potential drug interactions
Tricyclic antidepressants
Non-selective β-blockers

Maximum doses of lignocaine and adrenaline

In regional anaesthesia the maximum recommended safe dose of plain lignocaine is 200 mg. Because the addition of adrenaline delays local clearance of the lignocaine larger volumes can be tolerated when adrenaline is added so that up to 500 mg lignocaine can be used when combined with adrenaline. (*Note*: a 1% solution contains 1 gm/100 ml ie 10 mg/1 ml.) There is no generally accepted maximum for adrenaline that can be safety injected. Patients with ischaemic heart disease are considered to be at risk from the increase in cardiac rate and output that may result from adrenaline usage. The most widely quoted safe maximum dose for these individuals was empirically considered to be 200 μg subcutaneous adrenaline (New York Heart Association). In healthy adults 500 μg is quoted by some authors to be the maximum dose that can be safely injected. Others recommend 200 μg for both healthy individuals and those with ischaemic heart disease. This maximum for all adults has been adopted by this author, since it provides adequate anaesthetic volumes for all minor to intermediate skin surgical procedures and a large margin of safety.

Drug interactions with lignocaine anaesthetics and adrenaline

There is much written about the *potential* drug interactions with local anaesthetics. In practice this seems to be only a real problem with the adrenaline content of the anaesthetic and non-selective β-blockers or tricyclic antidepressants. However, inevitably it is possible to produce a list of *potential* drug interactions and these are therefore also discussed.

There is no reported drug interaction that precludes the use of plain lignocaine as a local anaesthetic (Table 4.6). There are many drugs reported to produce small changes in lignocaine levels when this is used to treat arrhythmias. There is little if any documented evidence that these are clinically relevant to the use of lignocaine for local anaesthesia. Instances where these interactions may be important include amiodarone, β-blockers, disopyramide and cimetidine, all of which slightly reduce lignocaine clearance. It is probably sensible to reduce the maximum dose (Table 4.1) used in patients taking these drugs who also have other lignocaine-toxicity risk factors (Table 4.4). Midazolam and barbiturates reduce lignocaine levels.

The inclusion of adrenaline does introduce potentially hazardous interactions in patients taking non-selective β-blockers or tricyclic antidepressants and adrenaline should be avoided in these subjects (Table 4.6). The smallest dose reported to produce an interaction with a non-selective β-blocker was 8 ml anaesthetic containing 1 : 200 000 adrenaline. Monoamine oxidase inhibitors and phenothiazines were previously considered to produce dangerous interactions with adrenaline. It is now accepted that this is not so and patients taking these compounds can be given adrenaline-containing local anaesthetics.

Reactions to anaesthetic injections

Allergy to lignocaine, an amide anaesthetic, is extremely rare but does occur and may present as angioedema, urticaria starting at the site of injection and shortness of breath. By contrast, allergy to the ester anaesthetics (e.g. benzocaine) is relatively common. There is no cross-sensitivity between these two groups. If a patient describes a previous reaction to a lignocaine injection it is important to consider all possibilities before assuming that the patient is allergic to lignocaine (Table 4.8). If allergy cannot be excluded, an alternative anaesthetic such as prilocaine (Citanest) can be used. This can be given plain or with the vasoconstrictor felypressin (Octapressin), a vasopressin derivative, which has less effect on the heart than adrenaline and can be used in patients taking tricyclic antidepressants (Table 4.6). Investigation of reported allergic reactions to anaesthetics can usually be carried out by an interested specialist but ultimately will require a test injection of anaesthetic given when resuscitation expertise and equipment are immediately available.

Table 4.8 Possible causes of reported adverse reaction after local anaesthetic injection.

Physiological, e.g. a faint

Reaction unrelated to injection, e.g. spontaneous or aspirin-induced urticaria, allergic reaction to rubber gloves or other agent

Reaction to additive (Table 4.2). Allergy to parabens or sodium bisulphite may produce immediate-type urticaria response or possibly eczematous changes around the site of injection. Allergy to these agents can be tested by patch testing

Reaction to adrenaline. Inadvertent intravascular injection of adrenaline is surprisingly common in dental practice, e.g. approximately 10% of inferior alveolar blocks are associated with intravascular injection of anaesthetics. Patients will report immediate tachycardia, sweating, palpitations

Allergy to anaesthetic agent. Requires investigation using patch, prick and intradermal tests. Each should only be done if the preceding test was negative. Intradermal tests should be carried out under the supervision of an anaesthetist

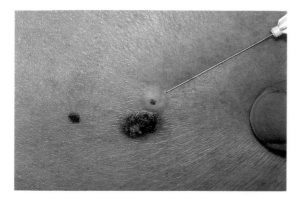

Fig. 4.2. Intradermal injection of local anaesthetic. The injection has been given too superficially in the skin producing a small wheal in the skin. This produces rapid anaesthesia but should be avoided as it is more painful than injecting the anaesthetic into the fat.

Method of delivery

Infiltration

Infiltration of the local anaesthetic into the skin around the lesion is the most widely used method. The solution should be injected slowly into the subcutaneous tissues to produce diffuse swelling of the skin. This takes several minutes to produce anaesthesia but is much less painful than injecting intradermally (Fig. 4.2). A variety of ways of reducing the pain of injection have been described (Table 4.3). Many are cumbersome and produce little benefit. In practice, a simple technique is to ensure that the patient is relaxed but prepared for the injection. Cooling the skin before injection may help. Use a long thin needle (e.g. 1½-in 27-gauge needle; see Appendix) so that a wide area can be numbed from one needle insertion. Distract the patient by rubbing the adjacent skin before inserting the needle; introduce the needle gently; inject slowly and only into the subcutaneous tissue. Reinsert the needle through skin that is already numbed and where possible start the injection as close as possible to the origin of the sensory nerve supplying that site. In children other simple and effective measures can be used to ensure success (Table 4.9). Your anaesthetic technique can be greatly improved by ex-

periencing the consequences of this approach when trying to inject yourself or asking someone to inject you with anaesthetic.

Table 4.9 Practical guide to giving local anaesthetic injections to children.

Apply EMLA cream 2 hours before starting
Give the child a mild sedative 1 hour before starting
Do not let the child see the needle
Use a 30-gauge needle (only ½-in long 30-gauge needles are available)
Distract by rubbing or squeezing adjacent skin before injection
Use 0.5% plain lignocaine rather than lignocaine with adrenaline. Follow up with lignocaine plus adrenaline if a longer anaesthetic duration is required
Inject slowly
Inject subcutaneously and wait
Only reintroduce the needle through numbed skin

EMLA, eutectic mixture of local anaesthetic.

Field block

When a large area innervated by several different sensory nerves needs to be numbed nerve blocks cannot be used. The area can be numbed using a field block, in effect infiltrating anaesthesia in a ring around the area, thus catching all sensory nerves entering the area. A long thin needle is helpful because it reduces the number of times the needle has to be inserted into the skin. Ideally, sufficient time must be allowed for the anaesthetic to numb each strip of skin so that the patient only feels the anaesthetic being injected and not the needle puncturing the skin (Fig. 4.3).

Nerve block

Large areas can be anaesthetized with little discomfort using small quantities of anaesthetic using nerve block techniques.

Supraorbital and supratrochlear block

The simplest nerve blocks are the supraorbital and supratrochlear block (Fig. 4.4) which result in a numb forehead and scalp as far as the vertex.

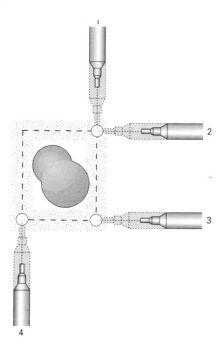

Fig. 4.3 Field block anaesthesia prior to excision; order of injections. The first injection is given subcutaneously. Warn patients that they will feel a needle and then a burning sensation as the anaesthetic is injected. Once the insertion site is numb advance the needle along one edge of the area to be anaesthetized, slowly injecting the anaesthetic. Choose the side closest to the origin of the sensory nerve innervating the area, with the aim of producing numbness distally prior to injection. The needle is then inserted at the next corner when numb, and the process repeated until a ring of skin around the target area is anaesthetized. A long thin needle is required so that the skin does not have to be repeatedly punctured. The anaesthetic must be given time to numb each strip of skin before the needle is reinserted, so that the patient only feels the anaesthetic being injected and not the needle puncturing the skin.

If the lesion is near the midline both sides should be numbed.

Mental nerve block

Mental nerve block (Fig. 4.5) numbs the lower lip and chin. When given via the mucosa the needle is aimed at the root of the second bicuspid or premolar (i.e. the 5th tooth) The position of the

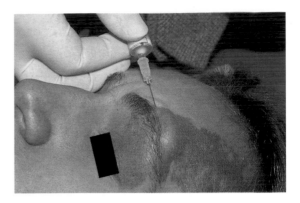

Fig. 4.4 Supratrochlear and supraorbital nerve block. The supraorbital foramen or notch can be felt along the orbital rim. The needle is inserted 1 cm medially to the origin of the medial and lateral branches of the supraorbital nerve, advanced down to bone just over the notch, withdrawn slightly, aspirated and 3–5 ml of 1% lignocaine plus adrenaline injected. The supratrochlear nerve leaves the orbit approximately 1 cm medial to the origin of the supraorbital nerve. The skin from the eyebrow to the top of the scalp can be numbed using this block but not the upper lid. In this patient infiltration anaesthesia of the lid was also required prior to laser therapy.

mental nerve foramen varies with age. In an adult with normal teeth the foramen lies midway between the upper and lower edge of the mandibular body below the second premolar, whereas in an edentulous adult atrophy of the mandible causes the foramen to lie nearer the upper edge of the mandible. Bilateral mental nerve block is usually required when operating near the midline.

Infraorbital nerve block

Infraorbital nerve block (Fig. 4.6) numbs the cheek and upper lip. This is potentially the most difficult of the three nerve blocks described. If only the upper lip needs to be numbed, just the gingival branches of the infraorbital nerve are blocked by injecting into the sulcus between the gingiva and lip mucosa above the incisors and canines.

Approximately 2–5 ml of 1% lignocaine plus

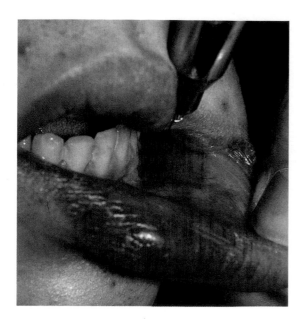

Fig. 4.5. Mental nerve block. The needle is inserted opposite the second premolar tooth and the needle advanced to the root of the tooth until bone is reached. Withdraw the needle a little. Inject approximately 2–5 ml of 1% lignocaine with adrenaline and be prepared to wait 10–15 minutes. The chin and lip on that side will be numb for 1–2 hours.

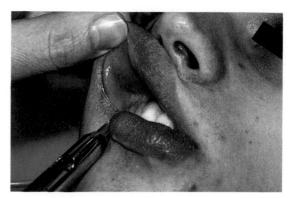

Fig. 4.6 Infraorbital nerve block. The middle finger is placed on the foramen and the lip held between the forefinger and thumb. The lip is retracted, the mucosa insertion site numbed and the needle advanced to the foramen until bone is reached. When the needle is correctly sited the swelling produced by the anaesthetic being injected can be felt with the tip of the middle finger. The foramen is difficult to palpate in an obese subject.

adrenaline is required and this produces numbness for 1–2 hours. In some patients it is difficult to palpate the infraorbital foramen. When the injection is given via the mucosa the middle finger is placed on the foramen and the lip held between the forefinger and thumb. The lip is then pulled away from the jaw, the needle inserted into the mucosa and a small quantity of anaesthetic injected to numb the injection site. The needle is then advanced towards the foramen until bone is reached. The needle is withdrawn slightly, the syringe aspirated and the anaesthetic injected. The swelling caused by the anaesthetic being injected into the tissues overlying the foramen should be felt by the tip of the middle finger. If this is not so the injection is being given in the wrong place and is probably going in too low. When injecting, ensure that the needle tip is below the orbital rim so that anaesthetic is not injected into the orbit. If this should happen the resulting oedema and haemorrhage will produce a range of alarming symptoms including blurred vision, diplopia, exophthalmos, loss of vision and pain in the eye, all of which should resolve spontaneously.

Ring block

Use 2% plain lignocaine. Fingers and toes are supplied by two dorsal and two palmar (plantar) nerves. The larger palmar digital branches, supplied from the median and ulnar nerve, run with the large palmar digital arteries. These nerves can be blocked by the injection of plain lignocaine into the base of the finger (Fig. 4.7). Because of the small risk of vascular compression caused by the injection of a large volume of local anaesthetic into the confined space bound by the skin and bone, no more than 3–4 ml of solution should be injected at a time into one finger and less into a small digit. To avoid this theoretical hazard some advocate injecting the anaesthetic more proximal at the level of the metacarpal head, i.e. just proximal to the distal palmar crease. This catches the common volar digital

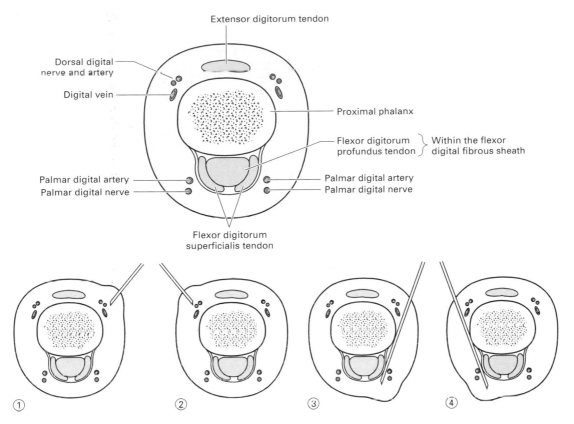

Fig. 4.7. Ring block anaesthesia. Use only 3–4 ml 2% plain lignocaine for a ring block. The needle is inserted in the finger at the position of 1.30 (1) and 10.30 (2) and a little anaesthetic injected to numb the insertion site. With the finger or toe grasped between the forefinger and thumb, the needle is advanced downwards on each side in turn, aiming for the tip of the operator's forefinger (3, 4). When the operator feels the tip of the needle under the patient's skin the needle is aspirated and anaesthetic injected as the needle is withdrawn. The process is repeated on the opposite side.

nerve and therefore numbs the adjacent sides of two fingers. It is also a much more painful injection. Practice suggests that this caution is more theoretical than practical as problems with digital blocks appear to be very rare.

Practice points

• Lignocaine anaesthesia is very safe. Experience suggests that the usual < 5 ml of 1% lignocaine plus adrenaline commonly employed is rarely going to produce serious problems in the absence of an idiosyncratic or allergic reaction, provided the drug is given slowly and care is taken to avoid intravascular injection.

• In all nerve blocks and particularly infraorbital nerve block, always aspirate before injecting because of the possible risk of intra-arterial or venous injection. This will produce acute overdose reactions and may also result in local anaesthetic being forced back along the vessel directly into the cerebral circulation.

• On the scalp inject the anaesthetic into the fat and not the subgaleal space (page 56). There are no nerves running in this potential space so the injection will not produce numbness.

• All nerve blocks take 10–15 minutes to take effect. Incomplete anaesthesia may occur due to anatomical variations and imperfect technique. There is no vasoconstriction of the numbed site and thus bleeding may hinder the surgeon.

• During nerve block anaesthesia the aim is to place the anaesthetic around but not into the nerve as this is painful and may damage the nerve. If the patient experiences shooting pains when the needle is inserted, withdraw the needle slightly (5 mm) aspirate and inject again slowly. Tingling in the innervated area indicates that the needle is near but not damaging the nerve, and the injection can be given. A needle with a 30° bevel and no cutting edge (e.g. spinal or retrobulbar needle) is best as this is less likely to cut into the nerve.

• The infraorbital or mental nerve block injections can be given both via the skin and the oral mucosa. The latter approach is much less painful.

• As some hand surgeons routinely use local anaesthetic with 1 : 200 000 adrenaline on fingers, it is highly unlikely that the patient will suffer any harmful effect if local anaesthetic containing adrenaline is mistakenly used on a digit. However, the aim must be to use only plain lignocaine on sites supplied by an end-artery, i.e. fingers, toes and penis.

Equipment

Using a dental syringe to deliver the anaesthetic is inexpensive and very convenient. If a self-aspirating dental syringe is used it is possible to ensure that the needle is not in a blood vessel before injection (Fig. 4.8). The long fine needles are ideal for skin surgery and because only one needle is used there is less risk to the operator of a needleprick injury. However, only 2% lignocaine with 1 : 80 000 adrenaline is available in the dental syringe vials and both concentrations are unnecessarily high for skin surgery. Dental syringe anaesthesia has been used for many years by dermatologists without mishap.

Disposable syringes have the advantage that almost any local anaesthetic can be used and large volumes of diluted lignocaine injected. Fine 27-gauge needles are available and should be used in preference to thicker shorter needles. 1% lignocaine with adrenaline, the solution most appropriate for skin surgery, is unfortunately only

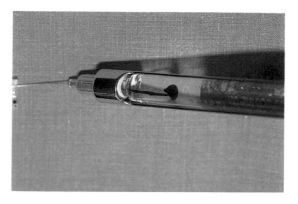

Fig. 4.8. Self-aspirating dental syringe. If a dental syringe is used, a self aspirating model should be selected. The dental syringe limits the choice of anaesthetic to 2% lignocaine plus 1 : 80 000 adrenaline. There does not appear to be any evidence that this very high concentration of adrenaline improves the duration or effectiveness of anaesthesia, compared to weaker solutions.

available in 20 ml multi-dose vials with their inherent risk of cross-infection (Fig. 4.1).

Eye anaesthetic

The conjunctiva and cornea can be numbed using topical anaesthetics agents including amethocaine or oxybuprocaine (benoxinate). The latter is shorter acting and stings less. Both are ester anaesthetics and should not be used in benzocaine-sensitive subjects (Fig. 4.9). The depth of anaesthesia depends on the number of applications because reflex tearing quickly washes the anaesthetic away. The patient should wear a protective eye pad for aproximately 30 minutes after oxybuprocaine instillation to prevent an unrecognized foreign body injury. Thus, the shorter acting oxybuprocaine is better than amethocaine since corneal sensation returns faster after the procedure. If a full thickness incision of the eyelid is required, the anaesthetic must be injected into both the skin and the fornix conjunctiva as the tarsal plate will prevent anaesthetic injected into the skin spreading to the conjunctival surface.

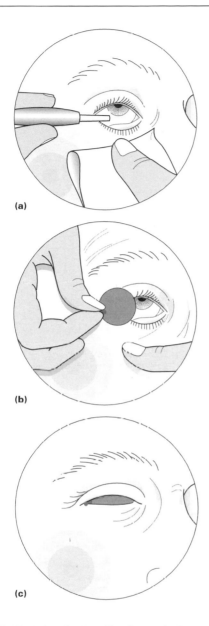

(a)

(b)

(c)

Fig. 4.9. Topical application of local anaesthetic eye drops. The iris conjunctiva is exquisitely sensitive. Eye drops should be dropped into the lower fornix, not on to the cornea. Pull out the lower lid, ask the patient to look up, drop the solution into the gap between the lid and the sclera (a). One to two drops are sufficient for each instillation, if more is used it will just run out. Adequate anaesthesia depends on the number of instillations rather than the amount dispensed each time. All local anaesthetic drops sting. A rubber eye guard designed for laser therapy (b) can be used to help protect against corneal injury (c) during surgery near the eye.

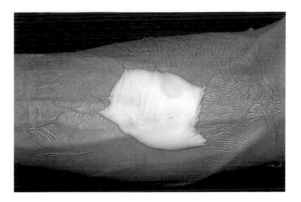

Fig. 4.10. EMLA cream application. It is important to use a large volume of EMLA cream and this can be held in place using a transparent adhesive film dressing (e.g. Opsite, Tegaderm) or clingfilm. EMLA should be left in place for a least 2 hours and removed just prior to surgery.

Using local anaesthetics in young children

Small local anaesthetic procedures can easily be done on small children, provided care is taken and an experienced nurse is available to restrain the child if necessary (Table 4.9). A mild sedative, e.g. promethazine, given 1 hour before will calm the child. If parents are present they should be seated where they can see and comfort the child but cannot see the procedure because of the risk of fainting. The skin can be numbed using a topical anaesthetic. For this purpose eutectic mixture of local anaesthetics (EMLA), a combination of lignocaine and prilocaine, can be applied under polythene occlusion 2 hours before the procedure (Fig. 4.10). The child will not feel the needle prick but will still probably feel the burning sensation as the anaesthetic is injected. Plain lignocaine should be used as this is slightly less painful than lignocaine with adrenaline. The child should not see the needle!

Further reading

Adrenaline use in local anaesthetics

Aitkenhead AR & Smith G, (eds) (1990) *Textbook of Anaesthesia* 2nd edn. Churchill Livingstone, Edinburgh.

British National Formulary (1995) p. 461. British Medical Association/Royal Pharmaceutical Society of Great Britain, London.

Kennedy WF, Bonica JJ, Ward RJ, Tolas AG, Martin WE & Grinstein A (1966) Cardiorespiratory effects of epinephrine when used in regional anaesthesia. *Acta Anaesthesiol Scand* **23** (suppl); 320–333.

Meechan JG, Jastak JT & Donaldson D (1994) The use of epinephrine in Dentistry. *J Can Dent Assoc* **60**: 825–34.

New York Heart Association (1955) Use of epinephrine in connection with procaine in dental procedures. *J Am Dent Assoc* **50**: 108.

Perusse R, Goulet JP & Turcotte JY (1992) Contraindications to vasoconstrictors in dentistry. Part 1. *Oral Surg Oral Med Oral Pathol* **74**: 679–686.

Nerve block anaesthesia

Eriksson EKG (1980) *Illustrated Handbook of Local Anaesthesia*, 2nd edn. WB Saunders, Philadelphia.

Scott DB (1989) *Techniques of Regional Anaesthesia*. Appleton & Lange/Mediglobe, Norwalk.

Stromberg BV (1985) Regional anaesthesia in head and neck surgery. *Clin Plast Surg* **12**: 123–136.

General texts

Auletta MJ & Grekin RC (1991) *Local Anaesthesia for Dermatologic Surgery*. Churchill Livingstone, New York.

Cawson RA, Curson I & Whittington DR (1983) The hazards of dental local anaesthetics. *Br Dent J* **154**: 253–258.

Covino BG & Vassallo HG (1976) *Local Anaesthetics: Mechanism of Action and Clinical Use*. Grune & Stratton, New York.

Henderson JJ & Nimmo W (eds) (1983) *Practical Regional Anaesthesia*. Blackwell Scientific, Oxford.

Howe NR & Williams JM (1994) Pain of injection and duration of anaesthesia for intradermal infiltration of lidocaine, bupivacaine and etidocaine. *J Dermatol Surg Oncol* **20**: 459–464.

Lawrence CM (1996) Drug Management in Skin Surgery. *Drugs* (in press).

Specific situations

Maloney JM, Lertora JJL, Yarborough J & Millikan LE (1982) Plasma concentrations of lidocaine during hair transplantation. *J Dermatol Surg Oncol* **8**: 950–954.

Rasmussen J (1982) Minor surgical procedures in children. *J Dermatol Surg Oncol* **8**: 706–707.

Thornburn J (1990) Factors modifying epidural block for Caesarean section. In: Reynolds F (ed.) *Epidural and Spinal Blockade in Obstetrics*. Baillière Tindall, London.

Drug interactions with local anaesthetics

Boakes AJ, Laurence DR, Teoh PC, Barar FSK & Benedikter LT (1973) Interactions between sympathomimetic amines and antidepressant agents in man. *Br Med J* **1**: 311–315.

Goulet JP, Perusse R & Turcotte JY (1992) Contraindications to vasoconstrictors in dentistry. Part 3, *Oral Surg Oral Med Oral Pathol* **74**, 692–697.

Stockley IH (1994) *Drug Interactions*, 3rd edn. Blackwell Science, Oxford.

Yagiela JA, Duffin SR & Hunt LM (1985) Drug interactions and vasoconstrictors used in local anaesthetic solutions. *Oral Surg Oral Med Oral Pathol* **59**: 565–571.

5: Haemostasis

Haemostasis is obtained by a variety of methods. Sudden vigorous bleeding in a small wound may be difficult to deal with without adequate suction (Chapter 2). Reassess your need for such equipment if intraoperative bleeding problems become frequent. Similarly, if postoperative bleeding complications regularly occur, reassess your use of postoperative pressure bandages. The management of patients taking aspirin and warfarin is discussed in Chapter 7. A completely dry wound is unnecessary and capillary ooze will be adequately dealt with by physiological haemostasis after suturing.

Vasoconstrictors

The vasoconstrictor effect of adrenaline (epinephrine) added to local anaesthetics prolongs the anaesthetic effect and has the added advantage of reducing bleeding. For these reasons adrenaline-containing anaesthetic should be used at all sites except the fingers, toes and penis. Only very low adrenaline concentrations are required and 1 : 200 000 adrenaline is quite adequate; higher concentrations are little more effective in prolonging anaesthesia or vasoconstriction. It must be remembered that the vasoconstrictor effect of adrenaline takes up to 15 minutes to achieve its effect, unlike the local anaesthetic effect, which occurs in the first 2–3 minutes.

The use of adrenaline may sometimes result in postoperative bleeding as constricted vessels start to dilate. It is thus important to ensure that haemostasis is correctly achieved with diathermy and pressure bandages are applied when necessary.

Physical methods

If all else fails, direct pressure will stop all bleeding in the short term, provided sufficient pressure can be applied. Postoperatively, pressure bandages are important and should be used routinely after extensive surgery (Fig. 5.1).

Vessels can be clamped and tied using a dissolvable suture. If a single large vessel can be identified, this should be clipped (Fig. 5.2) and tied off using a dissolvable suture (Chapter 6). Clipping the end of a small vessel using a pair of fine artery forceps and twisting may sometimes be sufficient. If a vigorously bleeding vessel within an area of undermined skin cannot be stopped, it may be necessary to expose the area further so that the area can be fully visualized.

If bleeding starts when a wound is almost fully sutured, this is commonly due to an adjacent vessel being punctured by one of the suture needles. Such bleeding normally stops when all the sutures are tied and pressure is applied for a few minutes to reduced local bruising. If bleeding continues, undersewing the area using a long needle may be successful. This will normally have to be sutured as an X centred on the bleeding spot. If this fails, the wound should be explored and the bleeding vessel identified and diathermied.

On fingers and toes a tourniquet should be used during surgery since adrenaline is contraindicated (Fig. 15.1).

Haemostatic dressings

Bleeding from open wounds (Chapter 19) can be readily stopped using an absorbable haemostatic dressing (Appendix) such as Surgicel (glucosic copolymer), Kaltostat (calcium alginate), Oxycel (oxidized cellulose) or Gelfoam (porous gelatin matrix). These materials may behave like a foreign body whilst dissolving in the wound and increase the risk of infection; it is thus best to remove large pieces before wound closure.

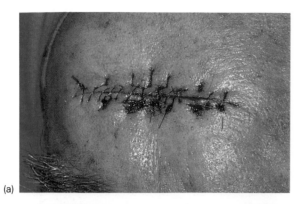

(a)

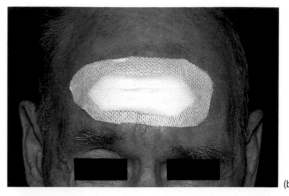

(b)

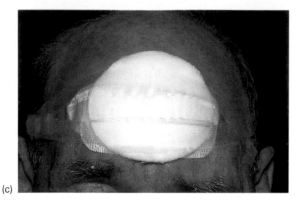

(c)

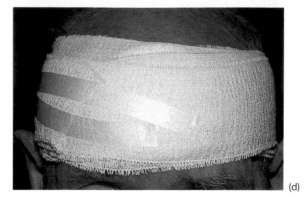

(d)

Fig. 5.1 Pressure bandage application. After excision of a basal cell carcinoma on the forehead (a), a smaller contact dressing was applied using a non-adherent dressing held in place with adhesive tape (b). The pressure bandage is applied on top of this. In this case two eye pads were used (c), and these were compressed using a 5-cm (2-in) crepe bandage (d). The pressure dressing can be removed by the patient after 24 hours. The wound dressing should remain in place until the patient returns for suture removal.

Within minutes of applying Surgicel, the white knitted fabric starts to fragment and, when saturated with blood, swells into a brownish gelatinous layer. It is gradually absorbed from the wound with little tissue reaction.

Such dressings can also be used in the management of a haematoma (Fig. 19.1).

Chemical haemostatic agents

Chemical haemostatic agents should only be used for wounds that are not going to be sutured, for example, after curettage and shave excision. These chemicals damage cells and should not be used in wounds which will be sutured as they leave dead tissue which predisposes to infection. Ferric subsulphate (Monsel's solution), aluminium chloride and silver nitrate are all effective haemostatic agents. Monsel's solution carries the risk of iron tattooing. Silver nitrate sticks are effective but caustic and, as they may produce scars, should not be used on the face (Fig. 5.3). Aluminium chloride (35%) in 50% isopropyl alcohol is an effective haemostatic agent, although this is not commercially available (Fig. 5.4). A 20% solution is equally effective.

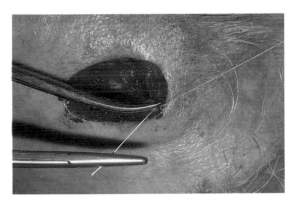

Fig. 5.2 Clipping blood vessel. A large artery, like this branch of the temporal artery, should be tied rather than coagulated. The vessel must be clearly visible; the absorbable suture should be sutured round the vessel and carefully tied.

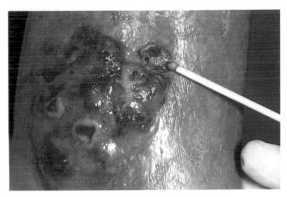

Fig. 5.3 Silver nitrate haemostasis. A silver nitrate stick is a very effective haemostatic agent but carries a small risk of scarring and thus should not be used on the face. It can be used to reduce granulation tissue or when taking a shave biopsy of a tumour. In this case the differential diagnosis was between overgranulating tissue or tumour. A shave biopsy was taken and bleeding stopped using a silver nitrate stick.

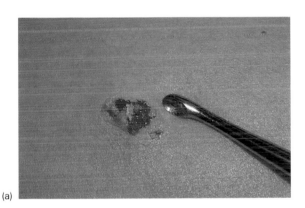

(a)

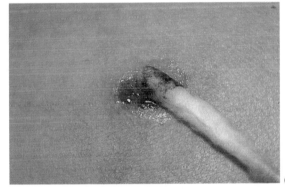

(b)

Fig. 5.4 Aluminium chloride haemostasis. After local anaesthetic injection this seborrhoeic wart was curetted off (a). Chemical haemostatic agents are only useful in oozing wounds and have no place in the management of vigorous bleeding. Wipe as much blood from the wound surface as possible and then roll a cotton bud soaked in aluminium chloride solution over the area and apply firm pressure (b). The blood changes to a brownish colour (c). Further application and pressure may be required.

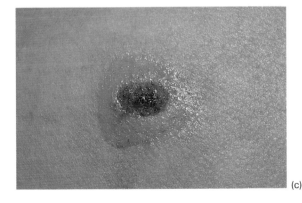

(c)

Electrocautery (syn. cautery, heat cautery, hot-wire cautery)

A cautery machine is useful for haemostasis after curettage and shave biopsy as it can also be used to destroy ragged edges or remaining fragments. It also has the advantage that the tip is simply sterilized by increasing the power; the tip briefly glows red hot, thus burning off any residual debris. The tip must not be glowing red when being used, as this risks melting the platinum tip. At best the expensive tip will have to be replaced; at worst, molten metal may drip on to the patient. When in use the power level should be set so that the tip is not glowing but is hot enough to char a cotton swab easily (Fig. 5.5). If the cautery tip drags on the tissue, as it is drawn across the wound, the tip is either not hot enough or being moved too fast across the skin.

Electrosurgery (syn. surgical diathermy, cold electrocautery) equipment

Electrosurgical equipment converts domestic alternating current into high-frequency alternating current which is converted to heat energy as it passes through a high-resistance medium such as

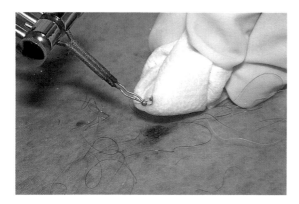

Fig. 5.5 Electrocautery. Mains-operated cautery machines are more expensive but preferable to the battery-operated instruments. The latter usually do not have a power control and tip temperature depends entirely on the level of the battery. The bead should be hot enough to char a cotton swab but not glowing red hot, as this may result in the expensive platinum tip melting.

the skin and fat. Different electrical waveforms produce tissue coagulation, desiccation or cutting. Some machines can produce all effects; others only produce desiccation. There is however some overlap between these effects so that the desiccation waveform, for example, can be used, albeit not perfectly, for cutting and coagulation (Table 5.1).

The other major difference between electrosurgery equipment is the way in which the machine electrodes discharge and collect the current. Monopolar electrodes produce current from a pinpoint source and complete the circuit via a large dispersive (neutral) electrode or plate attached to a distant body site, usually a limb. Bipolar electrodes produce and collect the current via a pair of forceps (Fig. 5.6). Monoterminal electrodes produce current from a point source; the current is not collected but dissipates into the patient. This type of equipment has the potential to produce high-frequency electrical burns caused by tiny sparks that cross between the patient and the operator. These can pass through a gloved finger and are similar to the static shocks sometimes experienced when getting out of a car. This only seems to occur when the machine is heavily used and the patient is lying on an electrically insulated couch. The spark occurs if a hand is removed from contact with the patient whilst the unit is being operated. This can be prevented by using a non-insulated couch or by keeping hold of the patient so that the charge trickles away from the patient via a large-area contact point and dissipates to ground via the operator or table.

For simple surgical procedures a monoterminal electrosurgical unit such as the Birtcher Hyfrecator is perfectly adequate and can be used for shave excision and curettage (Fig. 9.3). When this type of equipment is used, the tissue is either desiccated or fulgurized depending on whether the tip is touching or held slightly away from the skin. As the name suggests, when tissue is fulgurized, a spark jumps between the skin and the needle tip. The resulting heat causes superficial damage to the tissues. Electrodesiccation occurs when the needle remains in contact with the skin.

Table 5.1 Advantages and disadvantages of types of haemostasis.

Type	Uses	Advantages	Disadvantages	Electrosurgery equipment characteristics
Electrocautery (syn. cautery, hot-wire cautery)				
All types	Haemostasis after curettage and share excision. Cold point cautery of spider naevi	Simple, reliable Self-sterilizing Excellent for shave and curettage excisions Completely safe with pacemakers	Cannot be used for intraoperative bleeding Battery types may not have adjustable heat setting	
High-frequency electrosurgery (syn. diathermy)				
Monopolar (syn. unipolar) with dispersive (syn. indifferent, neutral, passive, return, ground) electrode	Coagulation or cutting	Reliable, safe	Expensive equipment Patient has to remove clothing because of earthing risk through metal components, i.e. studs, zips, etc. Dispersive (syn. neutral, indifferent, passive, return, ground) electrode or plate required	
Bipolar (Fig. 5.6c) e.g. bipolar lead on a Birtcher Hyfrecator or Ellman Surgitron	Coagulation	Reliable Safe No need to remove outside clothing	Forceps have to be sterilized	
Monoterminal (Fig. 5.6d) e.g. Birtcher Hyfrecator	Desiccation/fulguration	Fast Disposable sterile tips	Charring common Risk of high-frequency spark burns to operator and patient	

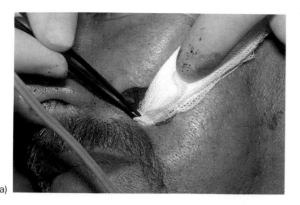

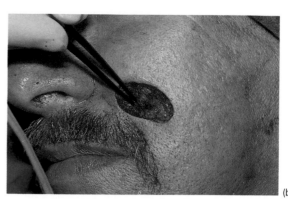

(a)

(b)

Fig. 5.6 Bipolar electrosurgery tip. With all electrosurgical equipment, haemostasis can only be achieved satisfactorily if the area being diathermied is relatively dry. Thus, bleeding points elsewhere may have to be staunched temporarily or blood removed using suction. The bipolar tip provides very precise surgical diathermy, produces relatively little charring and no earthing electrode is required. The forceps can be used to hold a cotton swab to dry the area to identify bleeding vessels (a) just prior to coagulation (b).

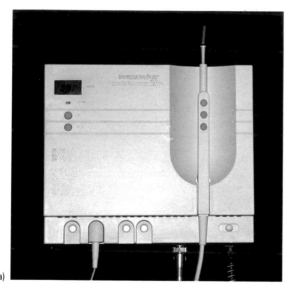

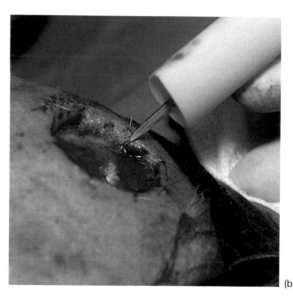

(a)

(b)

Fig. 5.7 Electrosurgical unit (Birtcher Hyfrecator). (a) This unit can be used for monoterminal diathermy, monopolar diathermy with a dispersive plate, and bipolar diathermy depending on the type of leads and forceps used. Disposable sterile monoterminal tips are available. If sterile handling is required, the hand piece can be sheathed in sterile tubing (b). Excessive use leads to charring. Whilst this generally has no adverse effect, infection rates may be higher, due to bacterial contamination of non-viable tissue.

No spark occurs and the depth of injury is slightly greater compared to electrofulguration. There is no effective difference in the type of tissue injury produced by electrodesiccation or fulguration; the only real difference is the degree of injury. Fulguration also results in tissue coagulation, albeit less effectively, i.e. with more charring, than a coagulating current could produce (Fig. 5.7).

Monoterminal diathermy can be made more precise if the bleeding vessel is picked up with fine forceps and the forceps touched with the electrosurgery tip.

Pacemakers and electrosurgery

There are no reports of pacemaker failure caused by dermatological electrosurgery, although this has been reported during prolonged monopolar diathermy of bladder tumours. The operator must be aware of this potential risk. Operating an electrosurgery unit near a pacemaker may either stop the pacemaker working temporarily, so that the patient's heart stops beating briefly, or cause the pacemaker to revert from a demand to a fixed rate pulse (the latter is not affected by the electrosurgical current). The effects last only as long as the unit is being operated. When diathermy finishes, the pacemaker reverts to normal function. Using any type of electrosurgical unit directly over the pacemaker may cause the pacemaker to stop. All demand pacemakers are at risk, although those made in the last 2–4 years are properly electrically shielded and less likely to be affected. All types of electrosurgical equipment, but not electrocautery, can cause the problem. Bipolar diathermy is least hazardous and should be used if possible. If any type of diathermy is used this should only be operated in short bursts (< 5 seconds), the patient's heart rate should be monitored and resuscitation equipment should be available. Diathermy should not be done within 6 in of the heart, the pacemaker or its leads. If monopolar diathermy has to be used the *path* from the active electrode (diathermy tip) to the neutral electrode must also be at least 6 in from the heart, the pacemaker and its leads. Monoterminal diathermy should be avoided, so if a Birtcher Hyfrecator or equivalent is used, preferably this should be used with the bipolar leads or, failing that, with a neutral electrode. Since each case is slightly different it is sensible to contact the patient's cardiologist prior to the procedure to discuss the nature and site of the surgery and the type of electrosurgical equipment to be used.

Further reading

Bennett RG (1988) Chapter 16 Electrosurgery. In: Bennett RG (ed.) *Fundamentals of Cutaneous Surgery*. CV Mosby, St Louis.

Boughton RS & Spencer SK (1987) Electrosurgical fundamentals. *J Am Acad Dermatol* **16**: 862–867.

Department of Health Medical Services Directorate (1994) *Evaluation*. Issue 211, May 1994.

Department of Health (1986) *Evaluation of Surgical Diathermy Units*. Health Equipment Information No. 153 May 1986. Available from the Medical Devices Agency (an executive agency of the Department of Health). 14 Russell Square, London, WC1B 5EP Tel 0171 972 8174.

(1978) Electrosurgical device interference with implanted pacemakers—a question and answer section. *J Am Med Assoc* **239**: 1910.

Larson PO (1988) Topical haemostatic agents for dermatologic surgery. *J Dermatol Surg Oncol* **14**: 623–632.

Sebben JE (1983) Electrosurgery and cardiac pacemakers. *J Am Acad Dermatol* **9**: 457–463.

6: Suture materials, suturing and knot tying

It is important to use the appropriate size and type of suture for each operation. The types of suture materials and knots used in skin surgery are discussed in this chapter.

Suture materials

Non-absorbable

Monofilament materials such as Ethilon, Prolene and Novafil (Table 6.1) produce less tissue reaction and hence less risk of stitch marks compared to braided silk (Fig. 6.1). The disadvantage of these monofilament fibres is their elastic memory, greatest with Prolene and least with Ethilon, which tends to cause the knots to unravel spontaneously, hence the need to tie square knots rather than a series of half hitches. By contrast, silk sutures do not unravel, however badly they are tied, and the cut ends are soft. Thus, silk is used on mucosal surfaces or where the suture ends may brush against adjacent structures. The major disadvantage of silk is the much greater tissue reaction and hence stitch marks. When the cosmetic appearance is important silk should not be used (Fig. 6.1).

Absorbable

Absorbable sutures are used to maintain the strength of the wound after the surface sutures have been removed, and to ablate deep dead space and reduce tension on the wound edge. The materials should thus retain their strength for as long as possible and whilst being absorbed produce as little tissue reaction as possible. Catgut and chromic catgut have relatively short maximum-strength life compared to the synthetic fibres (Table 6.2). They have little use in excision skin surgery. The new braided synthetic materials such as Vicryl and Dexon retain their

maximal strength for longer and are both relatively easily to use. Undyed subcutaneous sutures are preferable as the dyed suture is occasionally visible through the skin until reabsorbed. The monofilament absorbable suture material PDS (polydioxanone) has an even longer maximal-strength life. It is expensive but a very effective suture.

Subcutaneous sutures may extrude or spit through the scar before being absorbed if placed too high in the wound (Fig. 6.2). This usually appears 2–4 weeks after closure as an area of granulation tissue in the suture line. The suture should be removed if possible and the area allowed to heal spontaneously.

Needles

Suture needles should be handled carefully to avoid blunting the cutting point or bending the weaker end, or eye, where the suture material is attached. The needle should only be grasped with needle-holders in the middle third (Fig. 6.3). Needles vary in size, shape and cross-section.

Size

The aim is to use the thinnest needle and the finest filament the wound will tolerate, so that small suture holes are left with least risk of suture marks.

Needle thickness depends on the size of the suture material and the needle strength must be sufficient to withstand the pressures being applied to it. Different needle lengths are usually available for each suture size and the length required depends on the thickness of the tissue being sutured. The needle must be passed through the tissue at 90° to the surface and be long enough to be passed through the skin and then grasped by the forceps without damaging the

Table 6.1 Non-absorbable sutures.

Type	Material	Thread structure	Knots secure?	Available on drug tariff?	Tissue reaction	Colour
Silk	Silk	Braided	Yes	2/0, 3/0, 4/0	+ +	Black
Ethilon	Polyamide	Monofilament	Fair	3/0, 4/0, 6/0	±	Black, blue or undyed
Novafil	Polypropylene	Monofilament	Fair	No	±	Blue or undyed
Prolene	Polybutester	Monofilament	No	No	±	Royal blue or undyed

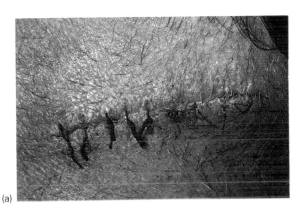

(a)

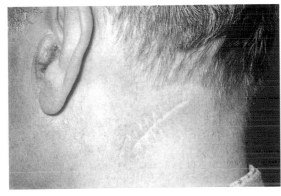

(b)

Fig. 6.1 Comparison of cosmetic result of silk and monofilament nylon sutures. This wound was sutured with silk at one end and monofilament nylon at the other. The sutures where removed at 7 days (a). The stitch marks at the silk-sutured end demonstrate the poor cosmetic result achieved from this braided suture (b). (Courtesy of Dr Peter Kersey.)

tip (Fig. 6.3). The jaws of the needle-holder must not be so wide that they tend to straighten the curved needle as it is grasped. If the needle starts to bend during use and has to be bent back into shape there is a risk that it will break. Loss of a piece of needle in the wound may greatly complicate an otherwise simple procedure.

Shape

Curved needles are exclusively used in skin surgery. The curve may be three-eighths, half or five-eighths of a circle or, in the case of subcutaneous sutures, shaped like a fish hook. The very curved needles can be placed in a confined space and are thus useful for inserting subcutaneous sutures. When using curved needles it is important to rotate the wrist when passing the needle through the tissue (Fig. 6.4). Simply pushing the needle into the tissue bends the needle out of shape, ultimately causing the needle to break.

Cross-section

Needles may be either cutting or non-cutting (round-bodied); the latter are not used in skin surgery. Cutting needles may have their pointed or cutting edge on the inner or outer curve of the needle (i.e. a reverse-cutting needle). The cutting needle has the disadvantage that the cutting edge points towards the wound so that when the suture is pulled centrally, the suture material is more likely to tear through the skin. By contrast, when a reverse-cutting needle is used the cut edge points away from the wound and the direction the suture is pulled; as a consequence there is less risk of the suture material tearing through the wound edge (Fig. 6.4).

Table 6.2 Absorbable sutures.

Type	Material	Duration at maximum strength (days)	Complete absorption time (days)	Available on drug tariff	Colours available
Catgut	Sheeps' intestine submucosa	7	Variable	No	Undyed
Chromic catgut	As above but tanned with chromic salts to delay absorption	10–14	> 120	Yes 4/0, 2/0	Undyed
Dexon plus	Polyglycolic	10–14	90–120	No	Undyed or green
PDS	Polydioxanone	35–45	180	No	Undyed or purple
Vicryl	Polyglactin 910	14–21	90	No	Undyed or purple

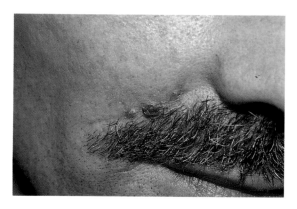

Fig. 6.2 Spitting sutures. The scar was carefully sited to run along the nasolabial fold above the patient's moustache. Two weeks later he returned with three small granulating papules placed at regular intervals along the suture line. These granulations were caused by subcutaneous sutures placed too high in the dermis. The suture may be removed from the granulation tissue or left to be extruded spontaneously.

Sterile skin closure strips

Adhesive tape strips can be used as an alternative to sutures, in conjunction with sutures, or after early suture removal. Tape strips do not mark the skin but, on their own, they do not evert wound edges to achieve the best scar. Adhesion of these strips can be improved by applying compound benzoin tincture BP (Friar's balsam) to the skin before strip application (Fig. 6.5). This should be painted onto the skin and allowed to become sticky before the tapes are applied.

Cyanoacrylate glue skin closures

Cyanoacrylate glue can be used for closing lacerations on hidden sites (e.g. scalp) and are particularly useful in children in these circumstances because they are painless. They cannot be used where there is tension, e.g. after elliptical excision, and are generally considered to produce less good cosmetic results than correctly used sutures.

Suture techniques

Knot tying

When using monofilament nylon sutures it is important to tie square knots because of the risk of the knots unravelling spontaneously. The technique is shown in Fig. 6.6. Practise this by attaching the suture to a seat arm or old pillow until it becomes second nature. If the knot starts to slip after the first two throws because wound tension is too great, make three throws, since this increases the frictional force required to unravel the knot, or kink the knot by pulling the suture endsin the direction of rather than at right angles to the wound (Fig. 6.6).

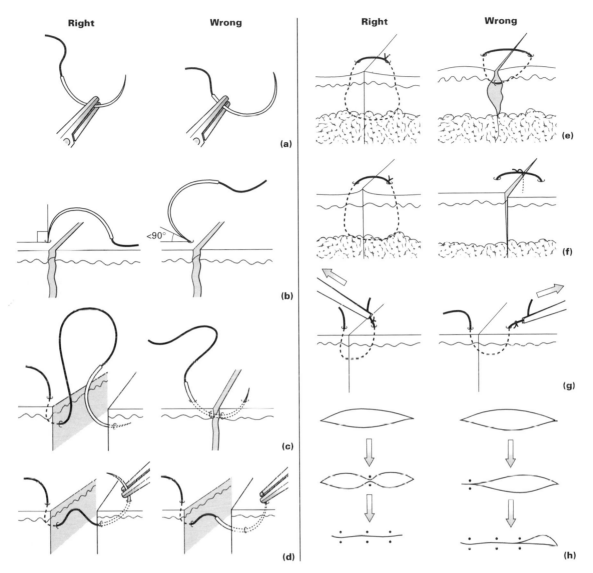

Fig. 6.3 Preferred technique during simple suturing. The needle should be grasped in the middle third, not at the cutting tip or the weakest part of the needle where the thread is attached (a). When the needle is pushed into the skin it should be at 90° to the skin surface so that the correct penetration of the skin occurs (a shallower angle of insertion will cause inversion of the skin edges); (b). Do not attempt to pass the needle through both sides of the wound in one movement. This may result in the needle tearing through the first side and makes the correct levelling of the suture difficult (c). When the needle is pushed through the skin, do not damage the sharp tip by grasping the point with the needle-holder until there is sufficient needle through the skin to allow it to be grasped at the correct place (d). Never use fingers to pick up the needle because of the risk of needleprick injuries. When designing a simple interrupted suture the skin edges can be everted by making the suture tract broader at the base than at the surface to produce a flask-shaped suture profile (e). Skin-edge eversion produces maximal dermis-to-dermis contact, thus enhancing healing. Ultimately the everted edge reverts to skin level as the scar contracts. If the wound edge is not everted at closure, contraction may produce a depressed scar. If the skin levels are unequal after the knot has been tied (f), the level may be slightly adjusted by moving the suture so that the knot lies on the low side. Failing this the sutures should be removed and the wound re-sutured (see Fig. 6.12). The knot should be away from a potential source of bacterial contamination, e.g. nose, not brushing up against a vulnerable structure, such as the eye, and towards the side with the best blood supply. The sutures should be cut approximately 5–7 mm long. If left longer they frequently become entangled in the next suture or the wound. Sutures should be removed after cutting by pulling the knotted end towards the centre of the wound and not away from it (g). Close an ellipse using the halving technique so that skin tension is equally distributed (h). Closure from one end may produce a fold of redundant skin at the end of one side.

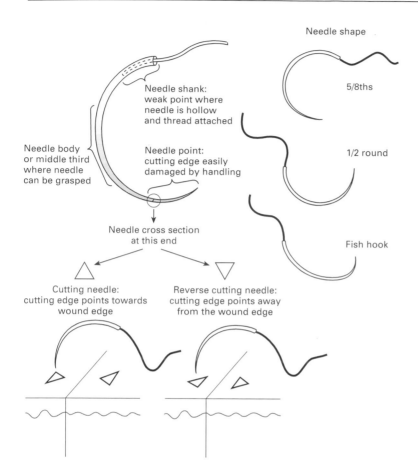

Needle shape

5/8ths

1/2 round

Fish hook

Needle shank:
weak point where
needle is hollow
and thread attached

Needle body
or middle third
where needle
can be grasped

Needle point:
cutting edge easily
damaged by handling

Needle cross section
at this end

Cutting needle:
cutting edge points towards
wound edge

Reverse cutting needle:
cutting edge points away
from the wound edge

Fig. 6.4 Needle shapes and types. A curved needle should be held in the middle third and not at the sharp point or the weak shank. Reverse-cutting needles are preferred because they produce a cut in the skin edge which is less likely to result in the suture tearing out when the suture is tied than a cutting needle. There are various needle shapes and lengths. The more curved needles can be placed in a more confined space. Needles bend when the operator mistakenly tries to push the needle straight through the skin rather than following the curve of the needle.

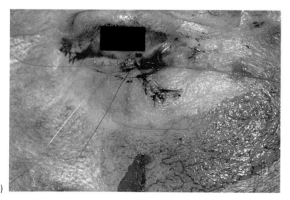

(a)

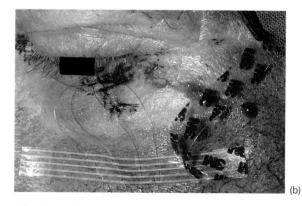

(b)

6.5 Adhesive tape strips. These can be used to strengthen a wound or to hold suture ends away from delicate structures. Tincture benzoin compound (a) or other skin adhesive can be used to give extra adhesion and this works best if it is allowed to dry slightly before the tapes are applied (b).

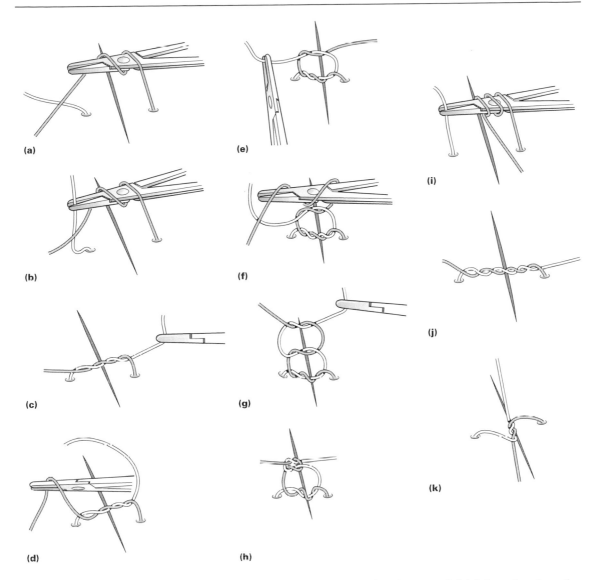

Fig. 6.6 Tying knots that do not slip. The first two throws (a, b) produce the first knot (c) which should appose the skin edges. The suture ends are pulled at right angles to the skin edges (c). The suture is then tied as a reef or square knot (d–g), which acts as a secure tie that prevents the first tie from unravelling. A gap can be left between the first tie and the reef knot to allow for skin swelling during healing (h). This will allow the first tie to unravel slightly but only as far as the reef knot. If the knot slips after the first tie, three rather than two throws increase the frictional force that has to be overcome to allow the knot to slip (i, j). Alternatively the knot can be kinked slightly by pulling the suture ends in the direction of the wound rather than at 90° to the wound (k).

Surface sutures

Simple interrupted sutures are adequate in most situations. They have the disadvantage that in larger wounds the skin edges may not be everted sufficiently, in which case the vertical mattress suture (Fig. 6.7) is preferred. This provides a deep and wide component that closes the dead

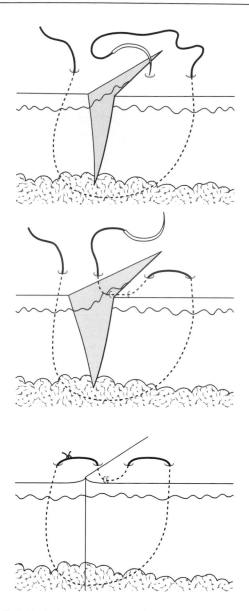

Table 6.3 Guide to suture size and time of removal with site.

Site	Suture removal	Monofilament suture size
Legs and back	10 days	3/0
Face	4–6 days	4/0 and 5/0
Elsewhere	5–7 days	4/0

Fig. 6.7 Vertical mattress suture. This useful suture everts the edges and eradicates dead space at the same time. Four puncture holes are created, so it is essential to remove the suture as early as possible when cosmesis is important.

the surface sutures to be removed in the shortest possible time (Table 6.3). A running or continuous suture is useful where there is little tension and the skin edges need to be apposed correctly (Fig. 6.8). It has the advantage of speed and economy. A combination of judiciously placed interrupted subcutaneous sutures, vertical mattress sutures at the centre of the wound and a running continuous surface suture are usually adequate for most wounds.

The running subcuticular suture (Figs 6.9 and 6.10) is a surface suture that can be left in the skin for a long time since only two potential suture marks are created. There must be little or no wound tension and, if present, this must be taken up using subcutaneous absorbable sutures and tape strips. Prolene is probably the best material to use as this slides through the skin very easily. The suture is difficult to do correctly, time-consuming and may be difficult to remove. If the suture breaks during removal the piece of mono filament nylon can be left in the skin permanently without causing any harm. Another problem with the suture is the difficulty in placing the suture correctly so that the skin edges are correctly aligned. Alternatively, an absorbable suture can be used and left in the skin to be absorbed. Thus, the suture is not brought out on to the skin surface but starts and finishes subcutaneously. The suture line tends to be bulky initially.

Subcutaneous sutures

Interrupted subcutaneous sutures should be placed in the skin so that the tension is taken by the dermis and the knot placed in the fat. In this position there is reduced risk of the suture spitting

space and provides strength and a close component to evert the skin edges. As with all surface sutures, stitch marks will remain if the sutures are left in place for too long. Skilful use of subcutaneous sutures and sterile skin-closure strips enable

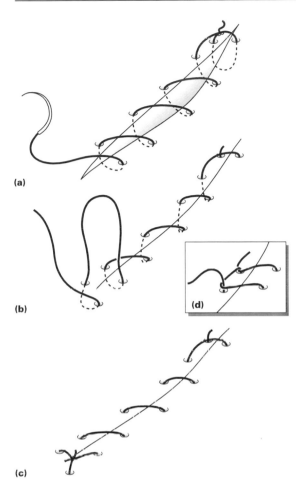

(a)

(b)

(d)

(c)

Fig. 6.8 Continuous or running suture. This can be used when there is no tension and the skin edges need to be accurately aligned. The suture should not be pulled tight as the wound edges will swell postoperatively. A simple suture is followed by repeated loops (a). The final loop is tied to the free end to secure to suture (b, c). A running locked suture (d) has the disadvantage of potentially causing greater suture marks but the advantage of holding the edges together more effectively whilst the suture is being tied.

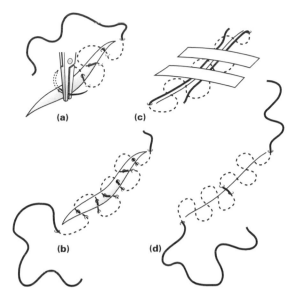

(a)   **(c)**

(b)   **(d)**

Fig. 6.9 Running subcuticular. The suture material, preferably Prolene, must be strong enough (i.e. 3/0 or 4/0) to withstand being pulled out without breaking (a). Before completing the closure, ensure that the thread runs smoothly through the skin when pulled from either end and note from which end it is most easily extracted. The suture ends do not have to be fixed or sutured into the skin as the suture will remain in place due to the frictional force of the curving thread (b). When the suture is completed and brought out through the skin, the wound can be further reinforced and the suture ends held in place using tape strips (c). The suture can be brought out on to the skin surface halfway along the closure if the incision is longer then 3 cm. This will help during suture removal as the suture can be cut or pulled at this point to reduce the length of suture that has to be removed in one go (d). The suture can be removed 10–21 days later. Alternatively, PDS suture material can be used and the subcutaneous suture material left in place, after cutting the ends off.

and adequate strength (Fig. 6.11). The suture should not be placed entirely within the fat as this will tear through when the suture is tied. If the wound requires several subcutaneous sutures, and if tying one prevents others from being placed, then site the suture material in the skin at the required sites, clip the suture ends using artery forceps to prevent the suture slipping out, but delay tying the knots until all the sutures are in place. Alternative subcutaneous suture designs such as the running subcutaneous and horizontal mattress suture can all be used if required but have no major advantage over correctly sited interrupted subcutaneous sutures.

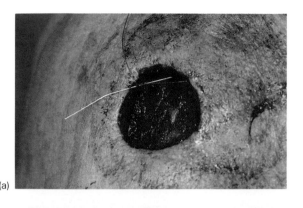
(a)

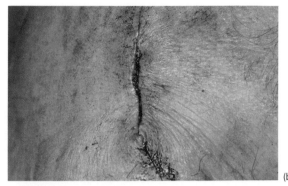
(b)

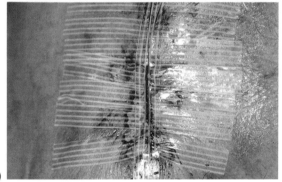
(c)

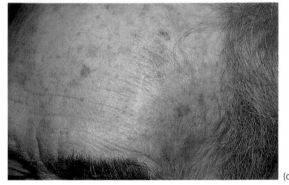
(d)

Fig. 6.10 Running subcuticular. A basal cell carcinoma was excised, leaving a large forehead wound (a). The defect was partially closed with interrupted subcutaneous sutures to remove skin tension. Vertical closure avoided elevating the eyebrow and the scar was designed to follow an oblique forehead crease. The dog-ear repair (Fig. 13.6) was performed as necessary to remove redundant skin at the tips of the closure. A running subcuticular Prolene suture was used (b). After checking that the suture ran freely through the skin, the ends were secured by first applying tape strips across the wound, then lapping the ends over the wound and holding them in place using more tape strips (c). The suture was removed at 10 days. The result was satisfactory (d).

Specialized sutures

Tip stitch

When suturing a skin tip into a corner the suture must be placed so as not to constrict the tip blood supply, as might happen if two surface sutures were used. The suture should run through the dermis of the skin tip but enter and leave the skin through the adjacent skin (Fig. 6.12a). This type of suture is used in complex repairs, such as when two adjacent dog ears are required, thus creating a W-plasty (Chapter 13).

Far–near–near–far (pulley) suture

If there is excessive skin tension, an ordinary vertical mattress suture does not always pull the skin edges together very easily. The far–near–near–far suture uses a pulley effect in that pulling one free end causes both skin perforation sites on that side to be tugged towards the centre. It can be used in thin eyelid skin but is of greatest use on the lower limb. Tension should never be so excessive that the skin edges are effectively is-chaemic. It is usually sufficient to place two or three such sutures in the centre of the wound and

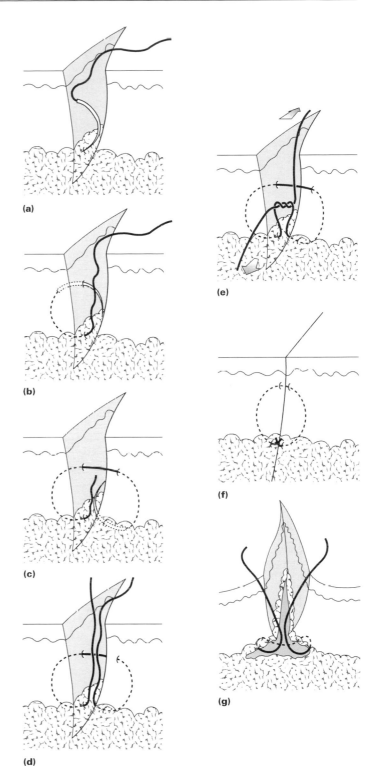

Fig. 6.11 Subcutaneous suture (buried interrupted suture). This important suture is designed to eradicate dead space and reduce tension, so that wound strength is still sufficient when surface sutures are removed. The strength comes from passing the knot through the dermis (a–d) but the bulk, i.e. the knot, of the suture needs to be in the fat to aid absorption (f). When the first two throws are pulled tight this should be done in the direction of the wound (e) in severe jerking movements rather than across the wound (compare with Fig. 6.6c). Subcutaneous sutures may produce inversion of the wound edges. This can be avoided by using a butterfly suture (g) where the bite through the dermis is sited further away from the wound edge and under the lower level of the undermined skin.

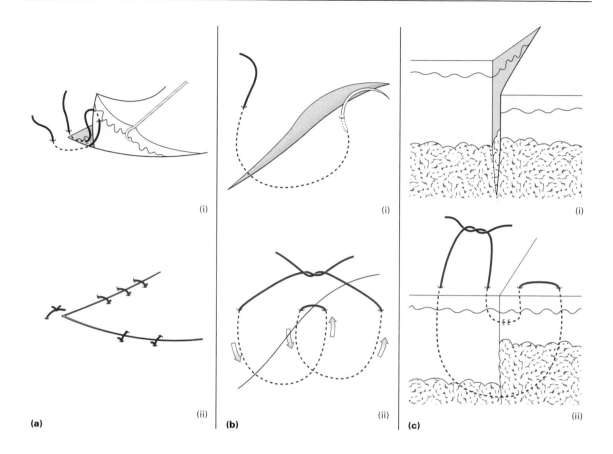

(i) (ii) **(a)**   (i) (ii) **(b)**   (i) (ii) **(c)**

Fig. 6.12 Specialized sutures. (a) The tip stitch can be used during more complex closures and avoids impeding the tip blood supply. (b) The far–near–near–far suture is useful for sites where tension is high. The levelling suture enables thick and thin skin to be sutured and still produce a smooth contour. (c) The levelling suture is used when apposing skin of different thickness

use vertical mattress or interrupted sutures to ensure that the skin edges are correctly everted (Fig. 6.12b).

Levelling suture

When suturing two skin edges of different thickness ensure that the sutures are sited at the corner level on each side so that a flat rather than stepped scar results. This is particularly common around the eye when suturing the eyelid and cheek skin (Fig. 6.12c).

Suture removal

Remove your own sutures when learning how to suture as it will improve your suturing technique dramatically. Sutures should be removed as soon as possible to minimize the risk of stitch marks. The suture should be grasped using Whitfield's or similar forceps, lifted and pulled towards (rather than away from) the wound, and the suture snipped and then pulled out (again towards the wound). Pulling towards the wound reduces the risk of pulling the wound apart (see Fig. 6.3g). The suture material is best cut using sharp pointed scissors. A number 11 blade or stitch cutter can also be used but both tend to jerk the suture and wound, with the inherent risk of injuring or splitting the wound. If there is any doubt about wound cohesion after suture removal the wound should be reinforced with tape strips.

These are best applied as sutures are removed rather than at the end of suture removal. This minimizes the risk of the wound splitting during suture removal.

Practice points

• Stitch marks are caused by using the wrong material, leaving the sutures in too long or tying the knots too tight. If silk has to be used and cosmesis is important, the sutures should be removed very early (3–4 days) to reduce the risk of stitch marks. Monofilament sutures rarely produce stitch marks if left for less than 7 days provided the knots are tied with the correct tension.

• Fingerprick injuries can be dangerous (Table 7.5). Do not pick up needles or guide them through the skin using fingers.

• Close the ellipse in halves to avoid redundant skin on one side of the wound (see Fig. 6.3h).

• If a running subcuticular suture is used in a wound greater than 3 cm long, pass the thread above the skin in the midline to create an additional point of retrieval during removal.

• When using subcutaneous sutures select colourless thread rather then the dyed alternative as this cannot be seen through the skin as the suture will persist for several months and may be visible under the skin.

Further reading

Bennett RG (1988) Chapter 8 Materials for wound closure. *Fundamentals of Cutaneous Surgery.* CV Mosby, St Louis.

Moy RL, Waldman B, Hein DW (1992) A review of suture and suturing techniques. *J Dermatol Surg Oncol* **18**: 785–9.

Stegman SJ (1975) Fifteen ways to close surgical wounds. *J Dermatol Surg Oncol* **1**: 25–31.

Stegman SJ, Tromovitch TA & Glogau RG (1982) *Basics of Dermatologic Surgery.* Year Book, Chicago.

Zachary CB (1991) *Basic Cutaneous Surgery: A Primer in Technique.* Churchill Livingstone, New York.

7: Preoperative assessment and preparation

Is treatment necessary and what is the most appropriate procedure?

Before contemplating surgery, a working or differential diagnosis is essential since this will determine the need for treatment, the type of procedure suitable and exclude inappropriate methods (Table 7.1). For example, seborrhoeic warts do not need to be treated; reassurance is frequently sufficient. If treatment is required, cryotherapy or curettage is simpler and produces potentially better cosmetic results than excision, which is inappropriate. By contrast, if a basal cell carcinoma is excised, a 3 mm margin is required; if curetted at least two cycles of curettage and cautery should be used and if treated with cryotherapy, two 30-minute freeze cycles (Table 18.1) are necessary.

Is the patient fit for the procedure?

General health and personality

The patient's general health and personality must be considered when contemplating local anaesthetic surgery. Will he/she be able to lie still for long enough? Is he/she able to lie flat? Is someone at home to look after him/her if something goes wrong after the operation? Does he/she have any other serious medical illness such as epilepsy or ischaemic heart disease that might cause problems during the procedure? The checklist (Table 7.2) covers most possibilities. The patient's temperament must also be considered as

Table 7.1 Considerations before surgery.

What is the differential diagnosis?
Is treatment necessary?
What treatments are available?
Which will produce the best result?
Is the patient fit for surgery?
What could go wrong?
Does the patient understand what is involved and the risks?
Are you prepared for emergencies?

Table 7.2 History-taking prior to surgery.

Allergic reactions
Antibiotics
Local anaesthetics
Topical antiseptics, e.g. chlorhexidine or iodine

Drugs taken
May cause bleeding problems: aspirin, NSAIDs, anticoagulants
May interact with adrenaline (Table 4.6): β-blockers, tricyclic antidepressants
May predispose to lignocaine toxicity (Table 4.6): amiodarone, β-blockers, cimetidine, disopyramide

General health conditions that may predispose to lignocaine toxicity
Renal failure, liver disease, heart failure

Previous bleeding problems
Bleeding problems at the dentist?

General health problems that may interfere with operation
Pacemaker fitted?
Need for antibiotic prophylaxis? (Table 7.3)
Epilepsy — risk of fitting during procedure
Diabetes — infection risk, potential for peripheral ischaemia, need to continue diabetic therapy, timing of procedure if taking insulin

Contraindications to adrenaline (Table 4.7)
Recent myocardial infarction
Unstable angina
Uncontrolled hypertension/diabetes/hyperthyroidism
Recent coronary artery bypass surgery
Refractory cardiac arrhythmias

Potential cross-infection risk
HIV and hepatitis risk factors

NSAIDs, non-steroidal anti-inflammatory drugs; HIV, human immunodeficiency virus.

some individuals are too frightened to contemplate being operated on whilst conscious. It is also important, particularly around the eye, to ensure that the subject does not mind the skin being manipulated at the proposed operation site.

Patients at risk from bacterial endocarditis

The need for prophylactic antibiotics to prevent bacterial endocarditis prior to skin surgical procedures is not established. Prophylaxis is recommended in dental and other surgical procedures where there is an established high incidence (> 20%) of transient bacteraemia. A lower threshold (5–10% incidence of transient bacteraemia) is considered appropriate for patients with prosthetic valves, who have almost twice the risk of developing endocarditis compared to other at-risk patients. There are few studies of the incidence of bacteraemia occurring during the course of skin surgery procedures. During curettage none of 22 cases had demonstrable bacteraemia. Procedures on eroded but not clinically infected skin lesions produced bacteraemia in 3% of cases. By contrast, manipulation of a staphylococcal boil resulted in bacteraemia in 38% of cases. There are anecdotal reports of bacterial endocarditis occurring after skin surgical procedures on infected skin. As a result it is considered prudent to offer prophylaxis when operations are performed through infected or potentially infected skin but not intact skin (Table 7.3). A wound infection arising in a patient with a prosthetic valve should receive prompt and vigorous treatment. As the anticipated organism is likely to be *Staphylococcus aureus* or *S. epidermidis*, the antibiotics suggested are different from those used for dental procedures.

Human immunodeficiency virus (HIV)-positive or at-risk patients

When faced with an HIV- or hepatitis B virus-positive or high-risk patient, non-surgical approaches to the problem should be considered. If surgery is essential then additional precautions must be taken to protect staff (Tables 7.4 and

Table 7.3 Suggested antibacterial prophylaxis prior to skin surgery to prevent endocarditis in patients with heart valve lesion, septal defect or prosthetic valve.

	Routine prophylaxis (patients with acquired or congenital heart disease producing valve damage)	High-risk prophylaxis (patients with prosthetic heart valve or previous endocarditis)
Procedure to be done through:		
Non-infected skin	No prophylaxis	No prophylaxis
Clinically uninfected eroded skin	No prophylaxis	*Prophylaxis advised*
Infected skin	*Prophylaxis advised*	*Prophylaxis advised*
Regimen suggested		
Non-allergic	Flucloxacillin 1 g orally 1 hour before procedure	
Penicillin-allergic	Clindamycin 600 mg 1 hour before procedure *or* erythromycin stearate 1.5 g orally 1–2 hours before procedure + 500 mg orally 6 hours later	

7.5). The risk of HIV infection being acquired after a single needleprick injection from an HIV-positive patient has been estimated to be only 0.13–0.5%, although the consequences are catastrophic. If health care workers receive a sharps injury from a high-risk or known HIV carrier they should remove the glove as soon possible, encourage bleeding and wash the area with soap and water. Professional advice should be sought. The potential benefits of prophylactic zidovidine are not established, although it seems reasonable that this should be offered, and if used, started within 2 hours and continued for 6 weeks. The worker should be tested at 3- and 6-month intervals to check for seroconversion.

Hepatitis-positive or at-risk patients

Needleprick injury from a hepatitis B e antigen (HBeAg)-positive patient carries an approximately 20% risk of acquiring hepatitis B.

Table 7.4 Infection risk in hepatitis B and hepatitis C patients.

HBsAg (hepatitis B surface antigen)	Anti-HBs (antibody to HBs)	HBeAg (hepatitis B e antigen)	Anti-HBe (antibody to HBe)	Anti-HBc (antibody to HBc)	Hepatitis C antibody	Infection risk	Comments
+	−	+	−	+*	−	High	< 0.001 ml of blood required
+	−	−	+	+	−	Low	Persistent infection
−	+	−	− or +	+	−	Non-infective	Past infection†
−	+	−	−	−	−	Non-infective	Immunized person
−	−	−	−	−	+	Low‡	

*May be negative in acute hepatitis B infection.
†Anti-HBc probably persists the longest and may be detected when anti-HBe and anti-HBe are both negative.
‡Lower infection risk relative to a HBeAg-positive individual but exact degree of risk is still unknown.
HBcAg is not helpful and is rarely tested for.

Approximately 1 : 500 otherwise healthy individuals are hepatitis B surface antigen (HBsAg)-positive/HBeAg-negative (Table 7.4). Needle or sharps injury from such a patient carries a much smaller risk of hepatitis transmission of 0.1%. Overall, the risk of hepatitis transmission from hepatitis carriers is 5–10%. A booster dose of vaccine should be given to previously vaccinated health care workers following a sharps injury from a known or high-risk hepatitis B patient. Non-vaccinated individuals should be offered active immunization with hepatitis B vaccine and passive immunization with hepatitis B immunoglobulin.

Table 7.5 Precautions to be taken in all local anaesthetic surgery.

Staff should be vaccinated against hepatitis B followed by post-vaccination serology (8 weeks) and booster vaccination (every 5 years)
Staff should cover any cuts and abrasions with waterproof dressings
Do not pass sharps hand-to-hand
Do not guide needles with fingers
Do not re-sheath needles
Dispose of all sharps in approved containers
Dispose of all clinical waste correctly

Additional precautions with HIV- and hepatitis B virus-positive or high-risk patients
Consider non-surgical therapy
Remove all unnecessary equipment and personnel from the operating area
Observe high levels of theatre discipline
Use double glove, high efficiency masks, eye protection, disposable gowns, boots
Disinfect operating floor and potential contact surfaces with hypochlorite solution

HIV, human immunodeficiency virus. Adapted from: Joint Working Party of the Hospital Infection Society and Surgical Infection Study Group (1992) Risks to surgeons and patients from HIV and hepatitis: guidelines on precautions and management of exposure of blood or body fluid. *Br Med J* **305**: 1337–1343.

Will the patient's medication cause problems?

Drug interactions

Potential drug interactions with local anaesthetics are listed (Table 4.6). Patients taking other drugs should be encouraged to continue therapy, especially angina remedies.

Patients taking aspirin or non-steroidal anti-inflammatory drugs

Aspirin and non-steroidal anti-inflammatory drugs (NSAIDs) inhibit platelet cyclo-oxygenase activity, resulting in altered platelet function and thus potentially enhanced bleeding (Fig. 7.1). Aspirin irreversibly blocks platelet cyclo-oxygenase activity, whereas NSAID inhibition lasts only as long as the drug is in the circulation. If possible, aspirin therapy should be discontinued at least 7

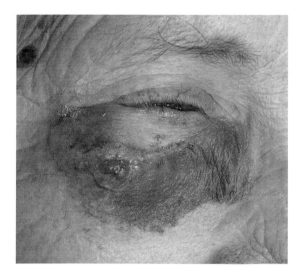

Fig. 7.1 Aspirin-induced bleeding. After injection of local anaesthetic, this patient developed striking subcutaneous bleeding. Further questioning revealed that she had taken an aspirin 2 days earlier. On the assumption that this extensive bleeding heralded potentially greater bleeding problems, surgery was postponed for 7 days, i.e. until the aspirin-induced inhibition of platelet function had resolved.

Table 7.6 Management of aspirin and non-steroidal anti-inflammatory drug (NSAID)-taking patients.*

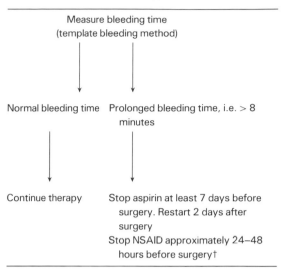

Measure bleeding time
(template bleeding method)

Normal bleeding time	Prolonged bleeding time, i.e. > 8 minutes
Continue therapy	Stop aspirin at least 7 days before surgery. Restart 2 days after surgery. Stop NSAID approximately 24–48 hours before surgery†

*Some advocate stopping aspirin in all patients.
†NSAIDs reversibly inhibit platelet cyclo-oxygenase activity. The effect persists as long as the drug lasts in the blood. Piroxicam and tenoxicam have the longest half-life of 70 hours, all other NSAIDs have a half-life < 24 hours, e.g. ibruprofen half-life 2 hours, naproxen half-life 15 hours.

days and NSAID therapy 2 days before surgery. If treatment is continued, approximately 15% of patients taking aspirin experience bleeding problems severe enough to interfere with the surgical procedure. Continuing NSAID therapy is even less likely to lead to bleeding problems. A recent study has shown that the 80% of patients taking aspirin or NSAIDs who have a normal bleeding time are not at risk from bleeding problems when therapy is continued.

Bleeding time is a reproducible method of monitoring aspirin-induced impaired platelet function. A pressure cuff (40 mmHg) is placed around the upper arm. The spring-loaded, disposable doubled blade is placed on the skin, usually across the arm, and the blade released. Two small linear cuts are created and the time taken for the bleeding to stop from these wounds is measured.

The blood flowing from the wound can be blotted using a filter paper but the clot must not be touched. The author recommends measuring the bleeding time several weeks before surgery is planned. If the bleeding time is prolonged beyond the normal range (2–8 minutes), patients are advised to stop aspirin at least 7 days before surgery. Agreement of the prescribing physician should also be sought in these instances. Patients who have a bleeding time within the normal range are advised to continue therapy (Table 7.6).

Patients taking anticoagulants

Before extensive surgery warfarin is normally stopped and heparin started in anticipation of briefly stopping this on the day of surgery. For small skin procedures it is frequently possible to operate without problems if the international normalized (blood clotting) ratio (INR) can be reduced to between 2 and 2.5. In some situations anticoagulants can be withdrawn for a few days prior to surgery without the patient being placed at risk. It will be necessary to discuss this with the physician monitoring the patient's anticoagulant control.

What local factors must be considered?

Infection risk

Operating through infected skin greatly increases the risk of wound infection. Crusted or broken skin surfaces are usually colonized with *S. aureus* and suturing infected skin results in a very high incidence of wound infection. Pre-surgery treatment with topical or systemic antistaphylococcal antibiotics is preferable to treating an infected dehisced wound subsequently. Alternatively, if surgery is performed on infected skin, the crust must be removed and the eroded area thoroughly cleaned with a detergent-based skin cleanser after local anaesthetic injection. The area should be cleaned again before surgery and a prophylactic oral antibiotic prescribed.

Anatomical considerations

The risk of injury to important local structures and anatomical features unique to the patient must be considered (Chapter 8).

Extent of disease

If tumour surgery is contemplated, ensure that the edges of the lesion are easily identified and that the correct margin of normal skin is included in the excision.

What to tell the patient before starting

Scarring hazard

Discuss the probable cosmetic results before surgery (Table 7.7). Use the word 'scar' in preference to possibly more soothing terms, as it is important that the patient realizes that a scar, however inconspicuous, is almost always inevitable. Be particularly aware when operating on keloid-prone sites or individuals (Table 7.8). The upper back, central chest (Fig. 7.2), breasts and shoul-

Table 7.7 Discuss the following possible long-term consequences.

Scarring
Loss of function — site-specific
Numbness
Tumour recurrence

Table 7.8 How to reduce the risk of hypertrophic or keloid scars.

Avoid operating in sites where keloids commonly form (Figs 7.2 & 7.3)
Avoid operating unnecessarily in people with a high risk of keloid formation — young people, African-Caribbeans
Design the wound correctly so that the scar runs parallel to the skin crease or relaxed skin tension lines
Reduce wound tension by undermining
Increase wound strength by using subcutaneous sutures if necessary

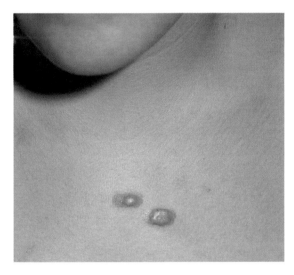

Fig. 7.2 Keloid scar. This young woman has developed two keloid scars on her chest wall at the sites of two chickenpox scars. Spontaneous keloids on the chest wall are common but also arise from acne folliculitis. Any injury at this site is likely to lead to further keloid formation.

ders are all susceptible sites (Fig. 7.3) and keloids are more likely to occur in young individuals and African-Caribbeans. Avoid any strictly cosmetic procedure in such patients and warn susceptible patients. If excision is essential in a predisposed

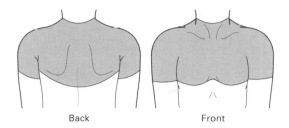

Fig. 7.3 Keloid/hypertrophic scar-prone sites. The upper back, anterior central chest, upper arms, shoulders and breasts are all keloid-prone sites. Avoid unnecessary procedures in these sites, particularly in predisposed individuals.

individual, use subcutaneous sutures as wound tension may be an aetiological factor.

Warnings of postoperative necessities

Patients may have the misconception that once surgery is finished they can go about their daily routine without problems (Table 7.9). It is surprising how often patients need to be told that they will need a bandage, their eye may have to be covered and consequently they may not be able to drive, they cannot go shopping, walking, jogging or play football immediately after surgery and will need to come back the following week for the sutures to be removed.

Table 7.9 Remember to discuss these potential immediate consequences.

Pain
Swelling
Haematoma formation
Tracking of haematoma
Eyelid oedema
Temporary loss of function:
   Directly related to the wound and dressing
   Due to anaesthetic paralysis of motor nerves (see
     page 12)
Need to rest
Sutures will have to be removed
A dressing may be required
The cosmetic result may not look good for a few weeks —
   avoid operating immediately before an important social
   occasion

Forewarn of immediate side-effects

Make sure patients are aware of the immediate consequences of surgery so that they will not be alarmed if they develop pain, swelling, temporary loss of function or bruising. It is also useful to warn patients with lesions on the face that they will look quite different for a week or so. Before surgery it is also worth mentioning to the patient that some numbness immediately around the scar is inevitable, although this can be expected to improve for up to 2 years after surgery.

Make arrangements for suture removal

Tell patients before starting that sutures will have to be removed the following week. This avoids the problem of patients telling you at the end of the procedure that they will be abroad when the sutures are due to come out!

Be prepared for emergencies

Patient collapse

Patients may faint even when lying flat. If this happens it is important to improve cerebral blood flow by raising the patient's legs or lowering the head to avoid an anoxic fit. Ensure that the foot of your operating table can be elevated and you and your assistant know how to do this. Other potential emergencies, including anaphylaxis, angina, cardiac arrest, respiratory arrest (usually only if intravenous sedative has been used) and epileptic fit, must be thought through before they happen so that you and your staff know what to do if these should occur. It is essential that you operate in circumstances where a suitably trained assistant can be called for in an emergency and appropriate resuscitation equipment is available.

Relatives collapse

Relatives frequently want to come into the operating room to give moral support or out of curiosity. If they are admitted, be sure to warn them that if they feel faint they must tell someone and sit down immediately. Even the most hardened individual may find watching an operation on a loved one very stressful.

Further reading

Carmichael AJ, Flanagan PG, Holt PJA & Duerden B (1996) The occurrence of bacteraemia with skin surgery. *Brit J Dermatol* **134**: 120–122.

Centers for Disease Control and Prevention (1996) Case-control study of HIV sero-conversion in health-care workers after percutaneous exposure to HIV-infected blood — France, United Kingdom and United States January 1988–August 1996. *JAMA* **275**: 274–275.

Haas AF & Grekin RC (1995) Antibiotic prophylaxis in dermatologic surgery. *J Am Acad Dermatol* **32**: 155–176.

Lawrence CM, Sakuntabhai A & Tiling-Grosse S (1994) The effect of aspirin and non steroidal anti-inflammatory drug therapy on bleeding complications in der-matological surgery patients. *J Am Acad Dermatol* **31**: 988–992.

Maurice PD, Parker S, Azadian BS & Cream JJ (1991) Minor skin surgery. Are prophylactic antibiotics ever needed for curettage? *Acta Dermato-Venereol* **71**: 267–268.

Recommendations for the Endocarditis Working Party of the British Society for Antimicrobial Chemotherapy (1990) Antibiotic prophylaxis of infective endocarditis. *Lancet* **335**: 88–89.

Recommendations of the Expert Advisory Group on AIDS (1990) *Guidance for Clinical Health Care Workers: Protection against infection with HIV and Hepatitis Viruses.* HMSO, London.

Richards JH (1932) Bacteremia following irritation of foci of infection. *JAMA* **99**: 1496–1497.

Sabetta JB & Zitelli JA (1987) The incidence of bacter-aemia during skin surgery. *Arch Dermatol* **123**: 213–215.

Scully C, Samaranayake L & Martin M (1993) HIV: answers to common questions on transmission, disinfection and antisepsis in clinical dentistry. *Br Dent J* **175**: 175–179.

8: Anatomy and danger areas

Excisions of skin lesions down to superficial fat will rarely result in exposure or potential damage to functionally important structures, except if the subject is extremely thin. Excision into deeper fat or down to deep fascia will result in exposure of important nerves and arteries and this is particularly important when large cysts or lipomas are being excised. This chapter will attempt to highlight areas where anatomical structures on the head and neck may be damaged by surgery. At all sites an important factor is the correct placement of the incision, parallel to the relaxed skin tension lines, so that the scar is not unnecessarily stretched (Fig. 8.1). The reader is referred to the excellent texts listed in the section on further reading for a description of anatomical sites not discussed.

Arteries of face

The head and neck blood supply includes extensive anastomoses. Thus, division of larger arteries during surgery will not result in ischaemic damage (Fig. 8.2). Larger vessels and other important structures can be avoided by hydrodissection (Fig. 8.3). This technique involves injecting saline into loose tissue below the lesion and thereby lifting the area to be excised off the critical structure before excision; the saline injection is delayed until just before excision and when the area is numb.

Veins

Venous drainage of the head and neck is similarly excellent and smaller veins can be tied and cut without compromising venous return. On the lower limbs, dilated leg veins are commonly encountered during excision surgery. When cut, both ends must be identified and tied with an absorbable suture. The external jugular vein runs very superficially as it crosses the sternocleidomastoid muscle. It may be easily damaged during superficial incisions on the neck at this site and may be difficult to repair (Fig. 8.4).

Lymphatic supply

Lymphatic vessels are virtually never seen during skin surgery. On the head and neck lymphatic supply to small areas can be temporarily disrupted

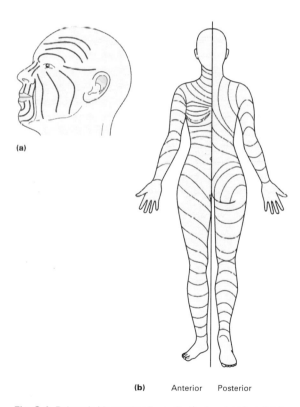

(a)

(b)   Anterior   Posterior

Fig. 8.1 Relaxed skin tension lines. On the head and neck (a) these are readily identified by following the existing wrinkle or skin-crease lines. On the limbs the lines tend to run obliquely around, rather than along the limb (b).

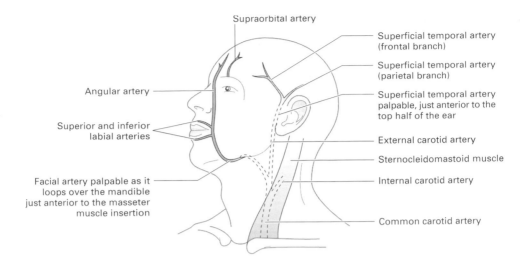

Fig. 8.2 Arteries of the head and neck encountered in skin surgery. The labial artery lies on the inside (mucosal) surface of the lip approximately 5 mm from the visible vermilion border. ---- = Arteries rarely encountered; ▬▬ = arteries frequently identified during superficial skin surgery on the face.

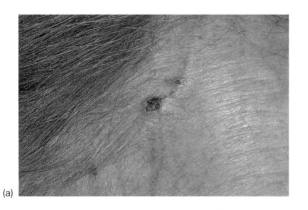

(a)

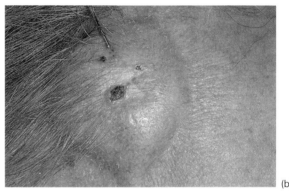

(b)

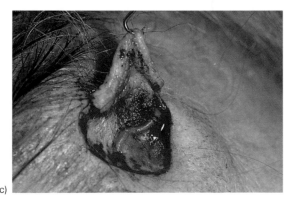

(c)

Fig. 8.3 Hydrodissection of skin tumours. This basal cell carcinoma was situated immediately over a branch of the superficial temporal artery (a). The tumour was lifted off this critical structure by injecting 10–20 ml of normal saline under the lesion immediately before excision (b). The tumour was then excised, leaving the artery in place (c).

Fig. 8.4 (*facing page*) Potential surgical hazard sites during skin surgery on the head. (a) Potential blood vessel and duct hazards; (b) potential nerve hazards; (c) potential cosmetic hazards.

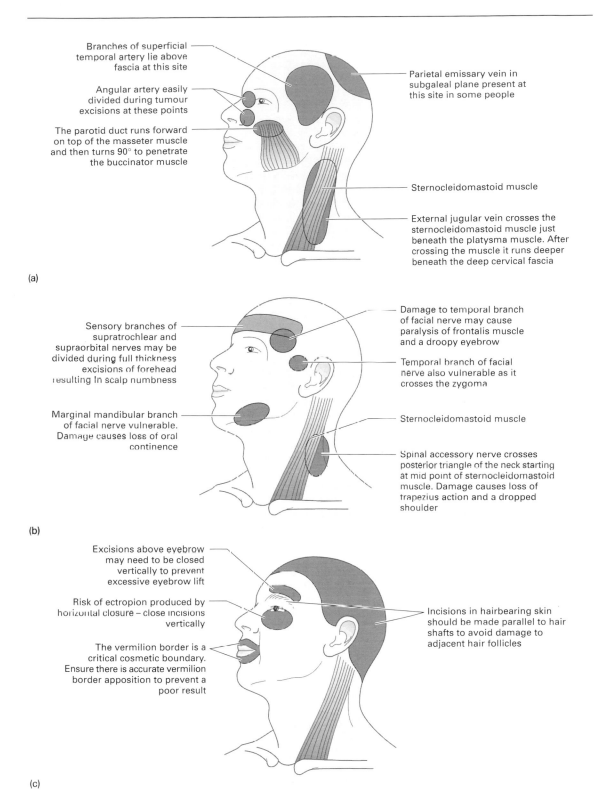

Branches of superficial temporal artery lie above fascia at this site

Angular artery easily divided during tumour excisions at these points

The parotid duct runs forward on top of the masseter muscle and then turns 90° to penetrate the buccinator muscle

Parietal emissary vein in subgaleal plane present at this site in some people

Sternocleidomastoid muscle

External jugular vein crosses the sternocleidomastoid muscle just beneath the platysma muscle. After crossing the muscle it runs deeper beneath the deep cervical fascia

(a)

Sensory branches of supratrochlear and supraorbital nerves may be divided during full thickness excisions of forehead resulting in scalp numbness

Marginal mandibular branch of facial nerve vulnerable. Damage causes loss of oral continence

Damage to temporal branch of facial nerve may cause paralysis of frontalis muscle and a droopy eyebrow

Temporal branch of facial nerve also vulnerable as it crosses the zygoma

Sternocleidomastoid muscle

Spinal accessory nerve crosses posterior triangle of the neck starting at mid point of sternocleidomastoid muscle. Damage causes loss of trapezius action and a dropped shoulder

(b)

Excisions above eyebrow may need to be closed vertically to prevent excessive eyebrow lift

Risk of ectropion produced by horizontal closure – close incisions vertically

The vermilion border is a critical cosmetic boundary. Ensure there is accurate vermilion border apposition to prevent a poor result

Incisions in hairbearing skin should be made parallel to hair shafts to avoid damage to adjacent hair follicles

(c)

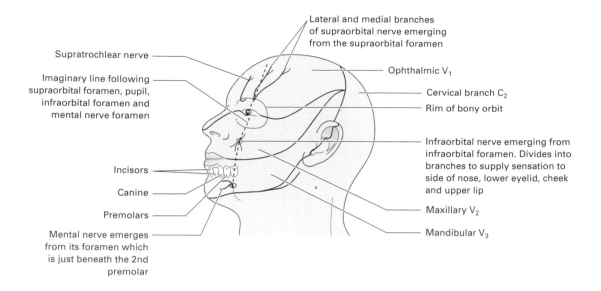

Supratrochlear nerve

Imaginary line following supraorbital foramen, pupil, infraorbital foramen and mental nerve foramen

Incisors

Canine

Premolars

Mental nerve emerges from its foramen which is just beneath the 2nd premolar

Lateral and medial branches of supraorbital nerve emerging from the supraorbital foramen

Ophthalmic V_1

Cervical branch C_2

Rim of bony orbit

Infraorbital nerve emerging from infraorbital foramen. Divides into branches to supply sensation to side of nose, lower eyelid, cheek and upper lip

Maxillary V_2

Mandibular V_3

Fig. 8.5 Sensory nerves to the face used in nerve block anaesthesia. Sensation on the face is served by the three main divisions of the trigeminal nerve: the ophthalmic, maxillary and mandibular divisions. Three important branches of these nerves — the supraorbital, infraorbital and mental nerves — emerge in the same plane along a vertical line running through the pupil.

by skin surgery, leading to local oedema which persists for several weeks. This is particularly common after extensive excisions under the eye, when swelling due to lymphatic blockage may persist for several weeks. Lymphatic drainage sites should be examined for metastasis during follow-up of patients treated for squamous cell carcinoma or melanoma.

Sensory nerves of face

Sensation to the face is supplied by the Vth cranial (trigeminal) nerve. The three divisions (Fig. 8.5) supply different areas of the face from the chin to the top of the scalp. The three important branches that can be readily used in nerve block anaesthesia (Chapter 4) — the supraorbital, infraorbital and mental nerves — all emerge in the same plane just medial to a vertical line running through the pupil (Fig. 8.5). These

foramina can be palpated by firm pressure as a small depression on the bone; greater pressure is painful. For this reason the foramina are easier to palpate on yourself than a patient.

The sternocleidomastoid muscle marks the border between the posterior and anterior triangles of the neck (Fig. 8.6). In the anterior triangle the carotid artery, larynx and other important structures run. In the posterior triangle three sensory branches of the cervical plexus — the greater auricular, transverse cervical and lesser occipital nerves — emerge from behind and then curl round to lie on the sternocleidomastoid muscle. These three nerves supply sensation to a large part of the neck and ear, and these areas can be anaesthetized by injecting anaesthetic along the posterior border of the sternocleidomastoid muscle approximately 2 cm above and 2 cm below a landmark called Erb's point. This point can be identified by connecting a line from the angle of the jaw to the mastoid process and then taking a vertical line from the midpoint. Where this line crosses the posterior border of the sternocleidomastoid muscle is Erb's point (Fig. 8.6). The accessory (XIth cranial) nerve emerges at the same site. This motor nerve lies deeper in the posterior triangle than the three sensory nerves and it is thus rarely affected by injection of local

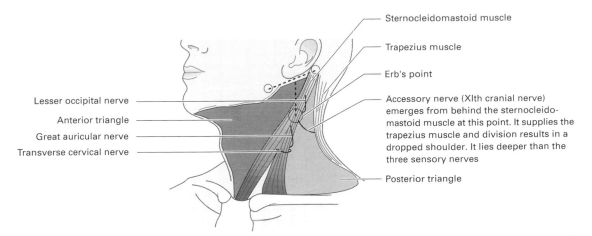

Sternocleidomastoid muscle

Trapezius muscle

Erb's point

Accessory nerve (XIth cranial nerve) emerges from behind the sternocleidomastoid muscle at this point. It supplies the trapezius muscle and division results in a dropped shoulder. It lies deeper than the three sensory nerves

Posterior triangle

Lesser occipital nerve

Anterior triangle

Great auricular nerve

Transverse cervical nerve

Fig. 8.6 A vertical line dropped from the midpoint of a line joining the angle of the jaw and the mastoid process crosses the posterior border of the sternocleidomastoid muscle at Erb's point. Alternatively a line drawn backwards from the top of the thyroid cartilage crosses the posterior border of the sternocleidomastoid muscle at Erb's point. The accessory nerve emerges from behind the sternocleidomastoid muscle at this point. Damage to this motor cranial nerve may occur during superficial surgery in the posterior triangle and results in paralysis of the trapezius muscle producing a dropped shoulder. Three important sensory nerves emerge from the posterior border of the sternocleidomastoid muscle approximately 2 cm above and 2 cm below Erb's point.

anaesthetic at this point. However, because it lies relatively superficially in the posterior triangle, it may be damaged during surgery, resulting in paralysis of the trapezius muscle producing a dropped shoulder.

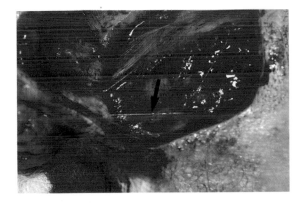

Fig. 8.7 Small cutaneous nerve. This small nerve was exposed during excision of a large tumour on the forehead. Nerves are more elastic and a shiny white colour compared to strands of connective tissue. An area of scalp numbness is likely to follow division of such a nerve.

Division of small sensory nerves (Fig. 8.7) frequently occurs in skin surgery and the consequences are rarely disastrous. The commonest problem encountered occurs after excision of a lesion on the forehead where the relaxed skin tension lines or forehead creases are at right angles to the direction in which the nerves run; thus these may be severed, producing distal numbness above the scar. Improvement in sensory loss can be expected for up to 1 year in most circumstances, as adjacent nerve branches appear to reinnervate the affected area.

Motor nerves of face

Motor nerves in the face supply the muscles which control facial expression and also serve the functions of eating, drinking and blowing. All motor supply is routed via the facial nerve. Two branches of the facial nerve are vulnerable during skin surgery — the marginal mandibular branch and the temporal branch (Fig. 8.8). These run superficially during part of their course and,

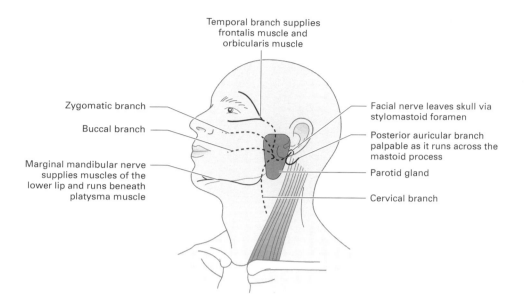

Temporal branch supplies
frontalis muscle and
orbicularis muscle

Zygomatic branch

Buccal branch

Marginal mandibular nerve
supplies muscles of the
lower lip and runs beneath
platysma muscle

Facial nerve leaves skull via
stylomastoid foramen

Posterior auricular branch
palpable as it runs across the
mastoid process

Parotid gland

Cervical branch

Fig. 8.8 Motor branches of facial nerve vulnerable in skin surgery. - - - - = Nerves rarely encountered; ▬▬ = nerves at risk during superficial skin surgery on the face.

unlike the zygomatic and buccal branches, do not share connections with adjacent branches to provide several innervation sources.

The temporal branch of the facial nerve supplies the frontalis and orbicularis muscles. The

Fig. 8.9 (*below*) Damage to temporal branch of facial nerve. Full-thickness excisions of the temple skin between the eyebrow and hair line commonly result in removal of the nerve supplying the frontalis muscle. This patient was trying to raise both eyebrows (a). Improvement may occur up to 1 year later and occurred after 4 months in this patient (b).

nerve to the frontalis muscle can be easily damaged during the excision of large tumours on the temple (Fig. 8.9). Here there is little tissue between the skin and periosteum and complete removal of an infiltrating tumour may result in removal of the temporal branch to frontalis, so that the eyebrow cannot be raised and the normal forehead furrows disappear. Orbicularis oculis is not affected because of the coexisting supply from the zygomatic branch.

The marginal mandibular branch innervates the orbicularis oris and lip depressors. Damage results in weakness of the lips with dribbling when eating and drinking. The nerve is vulnerable at the angle of the jaw as it emerges from under the parotid gland, since it lies very super-

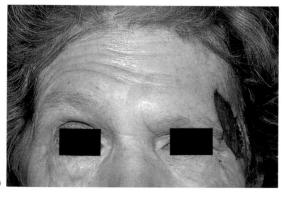

(a)

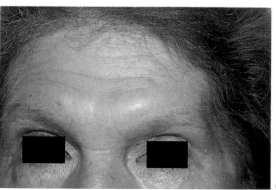

(b)

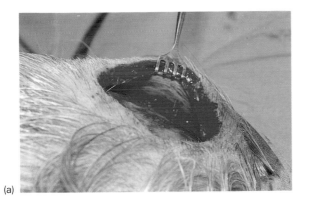
(a)

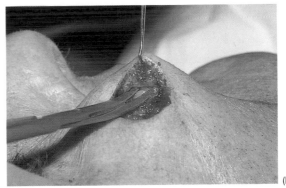
(b)

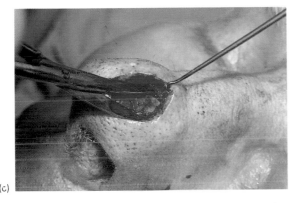
(c)

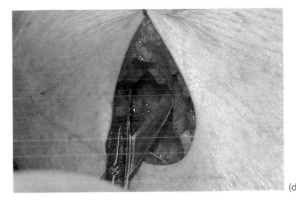
(d)

Fig. 8.10 Undermining levels. On the scalp (a) the avascular plane below the galea and above the periosteum should be chosen. On the forehead the equivalent level to the subgaleal plane is beneath the frontalis muscle. On the face undermine in the mid to high fat, although bleeding can be troublesome in the malar fat (b). On the nose the full thickness of skin down to periosteum is usually best, especially in people with thin skin (c). On the limb and on the trunk skin is undermined just above the deep fascia (d) or in deep fat.

ficially at this point. Anteriorly the nerve lies beneath the platysma muscle, so if this is visible its presence can be reassuring. The platysma is however frequently very feeble and is easily overlooked. The position of the nerve also varies with the head posture, so when the head is hyper-extended the nerve slides down below the lower border of the mandible. This drift downwards also occurs in older people without change in posture.

Undermining levels

Face

Undermining on the face can usually be done in mid-fat (Fig. 8.10). Injection of large quantities of very dilute local anaesthetic may aid the process (tumescent anaesthesia). Undermining must be done under full vision so that large vessels or nerves are not damaged. The latter requires careful time-consuming surgery and adequate lighting. An assistant and suction may also be required. The best technique is to tunnel into the fat with round-ended scissors, separating the strands of fatty tissue by repeatedly opening the scissors. An adjacent tunnel can be formed and the wall between the two trimmed carefully with scissors if necessary. Where possible, leave small vessels connecting the deeper tissues and skin intact, unless their presence impedes tissue mobility. Strands of tissue that are believed to contain a vessel can be diathermied with bipolar forces, before being cut to aid bloodless dissection. If undermining is difficult or results in excessive bleeding, this suggests that you are probably too high in the skin and undermining in the dermis. On the nose undermining is best done at a level just above the bone or cartilage (Fig. 8.10c).

Scalp

Undermining on the scalp is done in the subgaleal plane. The galea is the extension of the two layers of fascia that envelop the frontalis muscle on the forehead and the occipital muscle posteriorly. The galea (syn. galea aponeurotica, epicranial aponeurosis) is readily identifiable as a well-defined fibrous sheath. Immediately above it is the scalp fat, follicles and blood vessels and beneath lies a blood-vessel-free potential space. Beneath this is the periosteum and then the skull. Telling the difference between periosteum and galea may be difficult in the elderly when the galea may be quite thin. The galea is thicker and more mobile than the periosteum so that it moves easily over the underlying tissue compared to the relatively fixed periosteum. Furthermore, incision through the periosteum reveals the bony skull. The potential space beneath the galea (subgaleal space) is virtually avascular and blunt dissection at this level, i.e. above the periosteum and beneath the galea, can be extended for some distance with relative ease (Fig. 8.10).

Emissary veins connect the intracranial venous sinuses and scalp veins. As well as acting as a potential portal of entry for infections on the face to spread intracranially, these veins cross the subgaleal space. One such, the parietal emissary vein, not always present, carries venous blood via the parietal foramen from the superior sagittal sinus to the scalp venous system. This vessel may therefore be punctured when undermining in the subgaleal space over the back of the scalp (Fig. 8.4).

On the forehead the equivalent subgaleal space exists beneath the deep frontalis fascia; the forehead can be bloodlessly undermined at this level (Fig. 8.10).

Trunk and limb

Small excisions on the trunk and limb only require undermining in the deep fat. Larger excisions at these sites are best done by undermining just above the deep fascia (Fig. 8.10). In thin individuals this is relatively easy but in a fat person this may involve working down a hole several centimetres deep!

Specific facial sites

At certain sites it is also worth considering other structural factors that may be important. These include the lip, eyelid, hair line and scalp hair.

Lip

If an incision runs across the vermilion of the lips, the vermilion edge must be carefully marked to avoid a poor cosmetic result. This must be done before local anaesthetic injection because the vasoconstriction resulting from the anaesthetic may obscure the edge (Fig. 8.4). At this stage it is only possible to mark the lip edge by drawing with Bonney's blue. The latter may wash off and it is thus frequently necessary to duplicate these marks using a suture or by tattooing the vermilion edge with Bonney's blue; this will be completely resorbed in a few hours. When the lip is incised the labial artery may be cut. This runs in orbicularis oris muscle a few millimetres under the mucosal surface of the lip at about the level of the vermilion edge. If cut, both ends must be identified and tied.

Eyelid

Operating around the lower eyelid may result in ectropion if excessive downwards tension is applied to the lower lid. This is particularly a problem in the elderly who have lax lower lids with little tissue elasticity (Fig. 8.11). The amount of natural elasticity in the lid can be assessed by pulling the lid down and then releasing it. If the lid immediately snaps back into place, it is likely that a little tension or 1–2 mm ectropion imme-

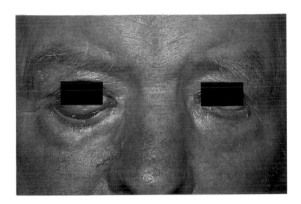

Fig. 8.11 Ectropion formation after skin graft on the right lower eyelid. Both lower lids show signs of senile ectropion, which is worse on the grafted side. Such a patient is particularly vulnerable. Others with apparently normal eyelids may have very poor lid tone. This can be assessed by pulling the lid away from the eye to judge how quickly the lid snaps back on to the sclera.

diately postoperatively will subside and natural tension will pull the lower lid back on to the eyeball. If, however, the lid does not snap back when pulled down, or only does so slowly, any procedure around the eye may result in ectropion. It is important to be aware that this may occur due to scar contraction, even when the immediate postoperative result apears satisfactory. In these circumstances the procedure should be planned so that the scar will increase rather than reduce eyelid tension. In most cases this means that excisions should be closed vertically rather than horizontally.

Hair line

If an incision goes across the hair line, ensure that the scalp margin is reconstructed so that smooth contour remains.

Scalp hair

If a hair follicle is cut through at the level of the root sheath, it may not survive. Because hairs grow obliquely through the skin, any incision through hair-bearing skin should be made parallel to the hair shafts, rather than vertically through the scalp, so that as few follicles are damaged as possible. When undermining on hair-bearing skin, ensure this is done below, rather than at the level of, the follicles.

Cosmetic units

The cosmetic results of surgery are better if the surgery can be designed to remain within one cosmetic unit. These units are recognizable areas, such as the nose, cheeks, forehead, etc. Each can in turn be divided into still smaller areas. Scars are also less obvious if they run along natural boundaries between cosmetic units or follow skin crease lines.

Local risk factors

Some of these have been mentioned before and the areas are summarized in Fig. 8.8. When operating around the eye, remember to use an eye shield if there is a risk of conjunctival abrasion (Fig. 4.9). It is always worth warning the patient of the potential development of a black eye (Table 7.9).

Skin tension lines and the orientation of scars

Incisions that follow the wrinkles or relaxed skin tension lines (syn. favourable skin tension lines, maximal skin tension lines) heal with a narrower and stronger scar line. These lines run parallel to the dermal collagen bundles and perpendicular to the direction of contraction of the underlying muscles (Fig. 8.1). On the face they are best identified by following wrinkle lines or asking the patient to adopt extreme facial expressions and on the limbs and trunk by manipulating the skin to find the direction of maximal wrinkling (Fig. 13.3). They are different from Langer's lines, which were mapped by observing the orientation of the ellipse produced after a circular wound was created in the skin of cadavers. Langer's lines should not be used for identifying the elective direction of excision, as these produce less good results when they do not correspond to the relaxed skin tension lines.

Further reading

Breisch EA & Greenway HT (1992) *Cutaneous Surgical Anatomy of the Head and Neck.* Churchill Livingstone, New York.

Kraissl CJ (1951) The selection of appropriate lines for elective surgical incision. *Plast Reconstr Surg* **8**: 1–28.

Langer K (1978) On the anatomy and physiology of the skin. I. The cleavability of the cutis. Translated and republished. *Br J Plast Surg* **31**: 3–8.

Larrabee Jr WF & Makielski KH (1993) *Surgical Anatomy of the Face.* Raven Press, New York.

Romain GJ (1986) *Cunningham's Manual of Practical Anatomy,* vol. 3 *Head and Neck and Brain,* 15th edn. Oxford Medical Publishers, Oxford.

Salasche SJ (1994) Surgical pearls: tips for scalp surgery. *J Am Acad Dermatol* **31**: 791–792.

Salasche SJ, Bernstein G & Senkarik M (1988) *Surgical Anatomy of the Skin.* Appleton & Lange, California.

Warwick R, Williams PL, Dyson M & Banister LH (eds) *Gray's Anatomy,* Churchill Livingstone, 37th edn.

9: Curettage

Curettage of seborrhoeic and viral warts

Curettage is only possible when the material being scraped off is softer than the surrounding skin, as with a basal cell carcinoma, or where there is a natural cleavage plane between the lesion and the surrounding normal tissue, as with a seborrhoeic wart. The resulting shallow wound heals by a combination of wound shrinkage and re-epithelialization from the follicular and edge epithelium.

Equipment

• **Essential:** lignocaine with adrenaline, curette (Fig. 9.1), haemostatic agent (Fig. 5.4). The curette must be sharp; various sizes (3–6 mm diameter is appropriate) and shapes (spoon or ring, e.g. Fox curette) are made. Blunt curettes can be sharpened. Disposable curettes are available (Appendix).
• **Optional:** electrocautery or electrosurgery unit (Fig. 5.8).

Indications

Seborrhoeic and viral warts (Chapter 16) can be treated by cryotherapy (Chapter 17) or curettage. The advantages of curettage are that the diagnosis can be confirmed histologically, a similar excellent cosmetic result can be expected and there appears to be a better chance of complete wart removal after one treatment of a seborrhoeic wart. The disadvantages are the additional time and equipment required by comparison with cryotherapy. Pyogenic granulomas and actinic keratoses are also commonly treated using curettage.

Viral warts

Solitary warts on the face of an adult can be removed by curettage. Warts at other sites that have failed to respond to other therapy (Chapter 17) can also be treated. Particularly difficult warts to curette off successfully are: (i) multiple finger warts that have not responded to other therapies; (ii) periungual warts, particularly if the warts have started to grow under the nail plate; and (iii) warts on the soles of the feet. These last type are discussed in Chapter 17. Genital and perianal warts may be treated with curettage if all other remedies fail.

Seborrhoeic warts

Multiple seborrhoeic warts are best treated by cryotherapy. Solitary warts or those that have not responded to cryotherapy can be curetted off if necessary.

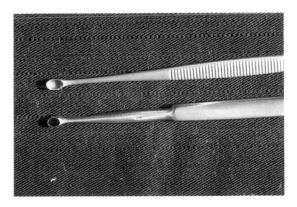

Fig. 9.1 Curettes: various types are available. A Fox ring curette (bottom) and Lang Steel double-ended scoop (top) are shown. The curette must always be sharp and small curettes are in general easier to use than large ones.

Technique

Numb the skin using the infiltration technique (Chapter 4). Tense and fix the skin around the wart using the finger and thumb. Scrape off the wart with the edge of a sharp curette using firm sideways scraping movements.

Viral warts

The technique is shown in Fig. 9.2. It may be difficult to get a plane of cleavage when curetting off a viral wart, particularly on mobile areas such as the lips, neck or genitalia. A cleavage plane can be started either by scoring around the wart using a scalpel blade or an electrosurgical unit (Fig. 9.3a). Scrape off any adherent remnants to leave a smooth surface and stop bleeding using either 35% aluminium chloride in isopropyl alcohol, cautery or electrodesiccation (Chapter 5). Do not use alcohol-based skin-cleansing solutions when

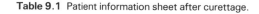

Table 9.1 Patient information sheet after curettage.

Your skin tumour has been curetted off. A small wound will remain which will take 2–3 weeks to heal over. The wound should be cleaned daily using cooled boiled water. Remove any debris or crust; apply a thin smear of antiseptic ointment and a small dry dressing. It does not matter if the wound gets wet in a shower or bath. After washing, clean the wound as before and apply a fresh dressing. If bleeding occurs, apply firm direct pressure for at least 20 minutes. Once healed, the scar may be red and slightly raised; after several months it will settle to a more flesh-coloured flat scar

using cautery or electrodesiccation because of the risk of fire.

A raw area a little bigger than the original wart will be left. The patient should be shown how to look after this and told that it will take 2–3 weeks to heal over completely. Initially the scar will be pink but will fade with time (Table 9.1).

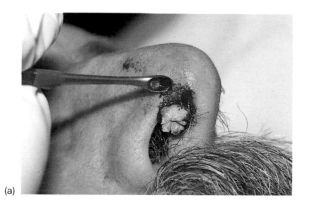

(a)

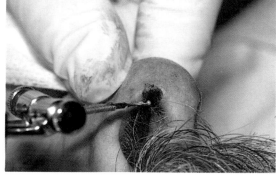

(b)

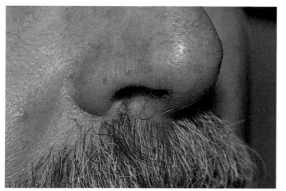

(c)

Fig. 9.2 A nasal viral wart: (a) during curettage; (b) after cautery and (c) 2 months later.

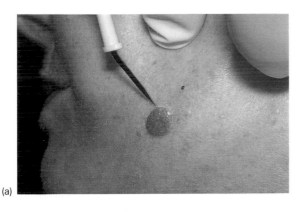
(a)

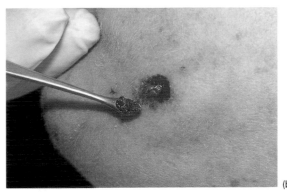
(b)

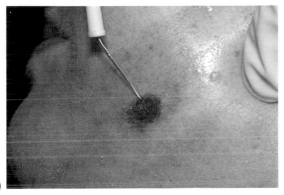
(c)

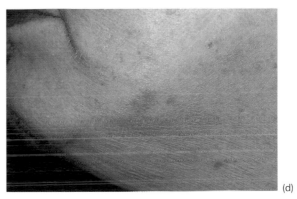
(d)

Fig. 9.3 Curettage of seborrhoeic wart on the face. The Hyfrecator was used to create a starting point for curettage (a) because a plane of cleavage could not be identified. The wart was curetted off (b) and haemostasis obtained using the Hyfrecator (c). This was the appearance 2 months later (d).

Seborrhoeic warts

Most seborrhoeic warts can be easily removed through a natural plane of cleavage between the base of the wart and the underlying dermis. If what appeared to be a seborrhoeic wart is difficult or impossible to curette off, it may be a warty pigment naevus, as these may appear identical. If necessary a plane of cleavage can be started by fulgurizing the wart edge using an electrosurgical unit (Fig. 9.3).

Curettage of basal cell carcinomas (BCCs)

Equipment

• *Essential:* local anaesthetic, small and larger sharp curette, electrocautery or electrosurgical unit (Chapters 5 and 11).

Indications

Curettage has been used successfully by dermatologists for many years to treat small BCCs (Fig. 9.4). At first sight curettage appears to be a simple technique requiring little skill or dexterity. The technique is fairly crude and simple but, without careful selection of cases and strict adherence to and understanding of the principles and limitations of the technique, recurrence rates can be distressingly high.

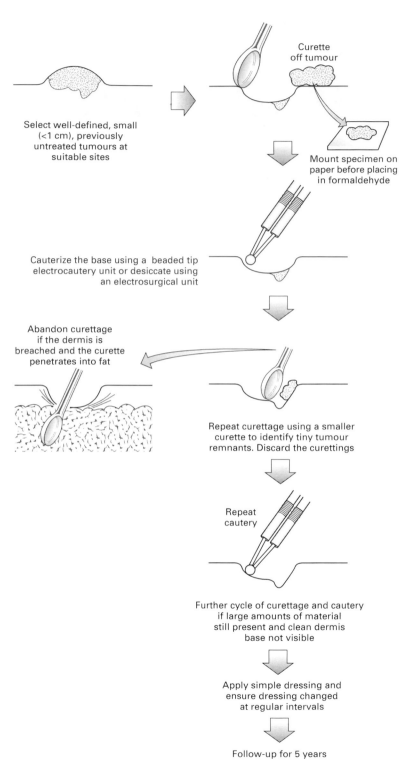

Select well-defined, small
(<1 cm), previously
untreated tumours at
suitable sites

Curette
off tumour

Mount specimen on
paper before placing
in formaldehyde

Cauterize the base using a beaded tip
electrocautery unit or desiccate using
an electrosurgical unit

Abandon curettage
if the dermis is
breached and the curette
penetrates into fat

Repeat curettage using a smaller
curette to identify tiny tumour
remnants. Discard the curettings

Repeat
cautery

Further cycle of curettage and cautery
if large amounts of material
still present and clean dermis
base not visible

Apply simple dressing and
ensure dressing changed
at regular intervals

Follow-up for 5 years

Fig. 9.4 Schematic illustration of the
stages of curettage and cautery of a
basal cell carcinoma.

Types of BCCs to treat

Not all BCCs can be treated by curettage and cautery. When correctly selected BCCs are curetted by experts, cure rates of over 95% can be expected. Worse cure rates result from the selection of the wrong type of BCCs (Table 9.2) or faulty technique.

Curettage of BCCs depends on the tumour being easier to scrape off than the surrounding normal tissue. Thus, any attempt to treat BCCs when strands of fibrous tissue separate clumps of tumour cells, e.g. morphoeic or previously treated BCCs, or when tumour cells have invaded local structures, such as muscle or fascia, will fail. Similarly, BCCs on sites where the skin tears easily, cannot be tensed fully or where hairs interfere with curettage should be avoided. The best results are achieved when small (< 1 cm diameter), previously untreated, well-defined, nodular or nodular-ulcerated BCCs are selected on sites where the skin can be held firmly and recurrence rates are low (Table 9.3).

Technique

Infiltrate the anaesthetic around, but not directly into, the tumour and allow the anaesthetic time to act. Tense the surrounding skin between the finger and thumb and scrape off the bulk of the tumour using a small, sharp curette. Blunt curettes are useless but the currette should not be so sharp that it is capable of slicing through the normal underlying dermis. The specimen pro-

duced should be sent for histology. Because this material is usually very fragmented it is best to mount it on a small piece of paper before dropping it in the formaldehyde (Chapter 21). Scrape off and discard any remaining tumour tissue. Carefully cauterize the entire wound surface using a hot-wire beaded tip or electrosurgical unit. This phase of the technique is designed to achieve both haemostasis and destroy remaining tumour cells. In the second cycle of curettage and cautery use a smaller curette to scrape off surface debris and use the smaller tip to search for residual tiny pockets of tumour. Much less tissue will be removed at this stage since the curette will be scraping against the normal dermis left after tumour removal. Cauterize the wound again. If a large amount of material is removed at the second stage, a third stage of curettage and cautery should be performed (Table 9.4).

The wound can be dressed using an antiseptic ointment and simple non-adherent dressing. The

Table 9.3 Sites to avoid when using curettage and cautery to treat basal cell carcinomas.

Sites with a high recurrence rate after all treatment modalities	Sites where curettage is technically difficult	Sites associated with poor cosmesis after curettage
Nasolabial fold	Lips	Vermilion border
Around the eye	Eyelid	Alar rim
Around the ear	Hair-bearing scalp	Nose tip
Scalp		Chin
Nose		

Table 9.2 Types of basal cell carcinoma (BCC) not to treat by curettage.

Large tumours: > 1 cm diameter
Tumours at sites where curettage produces a poor cosmetic result, is technically difficult or associated with a high risk of recurrence (Table 9.3)
Morphoeic, infiltrating or basi-squamous BCCs
Recurrent tumours
Ill-defined tumours
Tumours penetrating muscle, fat, bone, etc.

Table 9.4 Basal cell carcinoma (BCC) curettage technique.

Treat only small (< 1 cm), well-defined, nodular, previously untreated BCCs at suitable sites
Curette thoroughly using a sharp curette
Cauterize the base
Repeat the curettage using a smaller curette
Repeat the cautery
Abandon the technique if the dermis is breached
Consider the need for a third cycle of curettage and cautery
Follow the patient up yearly for 5 years

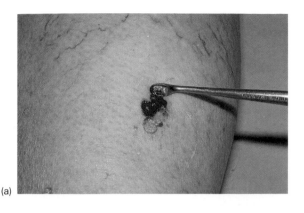

(a)

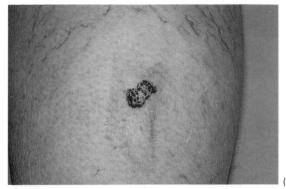

(b)

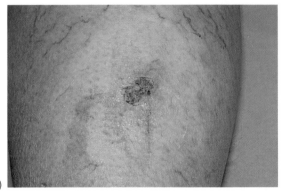

(c)

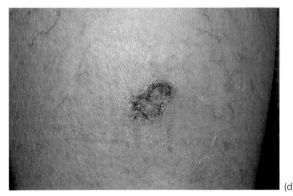

(d)

Fig. 9.5 Curettage of Bowen's disease on the lower leg. The area of involved skin can be scraped off easily (a), leaving a clean dermal base (b). If the dermis is punctured at this stage down to subcutaneous fat, curettage should be abandoned and the area excised. Bleeding is stopped by electrodesiccation or cautery (c). A second cycle of curettage and cautery may be necessary. Seven days later a crusted wound remains (d). The result at 4 months is good.

When selecting patients with lower-limb Bowen's disease for treatment by curettage or cryotherapy, remember that healing is greatly delayed by the presence of dependent oedema or an impaired peripheral circulation. In these circumstances other or no treatment may be more appropriate. Alternatively, dependent oedema can be controlled before and after surgery by suitable elasticated bandages.

dressing should be changed at regular intervals so that the wound remains clean and infection-free. A 10-mm BCC curette site will take between 14 and 21 days to heal and will produce a red and sometimes initially hypertrophic scar, which will flatten with time.

The patient should ideally be followed up yearly for approximately 5 years for signs of recurrence. If there is a recurrence the patient should be referred for other treatment. Do not attempt to curette off a recurrent BCC because the failure rate is very high.

Practice points

• Curetted specimens will be fragmented and will not include the whole of the lesion or show its attachment to the surrounding skin. If good histological material is required, either do not curette the lesion or do a small shave biopsy before curetting the bulk of the lesion.

• Do not be surprised if the histology report comes back with the comment 'incompletely excised BCC'. By the very nature of the specimen it will have tumour up to the edge. Good communication with the pathologist and making it clear that the tissue is a curetted specimen on the histology form will avoid this potentially worrying type of report. Curetted specimens provide a cytological diagnosis only; they give no information about the adequacy of the therapy.

• If at any stage during curettage the curette penetrates the dermis and enters the fat, the technique must be abandoned because it will be impossible to distinguish between the softer tumour tissue and the underlying fat. If this happens the curetted area should be excised down to and including fat.

Curettage of Bowen's disease

Indications

Intraepidermal carcinoma (Bowen's disease) is common on the lower leg of women. Discrete lesions can be treated by excision, cryotherapy, radiotherapy or curettage and multiple lesions treated using topical 5-fluorouracil (see page 122). Wounds on the lower leg heal badly, particularly if there is coexisting oedema or poor peripheral circulation. Curettage is no exception but may be a successful method as the amount of injury required to remove the area of affected skin is readily determined by the operator.

Technique

The method (Fig. 9.5) is similar to that used for the treatment of BCC. Care must be taken not to puncture the dermis as this will mean that the technique must be abandoned and the area excised.

Further reading

Bennett RG (1988) Chapter 15 Curettage. In: *Fundamentals of Cutaneous Surgery.* CV Mosby, St Louis.

Comaish JS (1986) Dermatological surgery. In: Verbov J (ed.) *New Clinical Applications, Dermatology. Dermatological Surgery.* MTP Press, Lancaster.

Kopf AW, Bart RS, Schrager D, Lazar M & Popkin GL (1977) Curettage-electrodesiccation treatment of basal cell carcinoma. *Arch Dermatol* **113**: 439–443.

Salasche SJ (1983) Curettage and electrodesiccation in the treatment of mid-facial basal cell epithelioma. *J Am Acad Dermatol* **8**: 496–503.

Spiller WF & Spiller RF (1984) Treatment of basal cell carcinoma by curettage and electrodesiccation. *J Am Acad Dermatol* **11**: 808–814.

Sweet RD (1963) The treatment of basal cell carcinoma by curettage. *Br J Dermatol* **75**: 137–148.

10: Snip excision

Snip excision is a simple and effective way of removing tiny skin tags and larger pedunculated skin polyps.

Equipment

- **Essential:** sharp scissors, forceps.
- **Optional:** haemostatic agent or electrocautery, local anaesthetic.

Indications

Skin tags

Skin tags are tiny harmless fibroepithelial polyps commonly seen around the neck and in the axillae and groins. They are small soft, non-keratotic, pedunculated, flesh-coloured or slightly pigmented tags. Some have the histological features of small naevi.

Large fibroepithelial polyps

Large polyps are usually solitary fibroepitheliomas, although old pedunculated moles, neurofibromata or fibromas may appear similar. Larger polps can be removed by tying a length of cotton around the neck of the polyp to occlude the blood supply. This method is certainly easier for the doctor but would appear to be more inconvenient and painful for the patient, and no histological specimen is obtained. Sending a tag that has dropped off using this technique will produce the alarming report of a haemorrhagic infarcted lesion, often with the caution that malignancy cannot be excluded.

Technique

Skin tags

Neck and axilla tags can simply be removed by snipping them off with a pair of sharp fine scissors (Table 10.1). Local anaesthetic is unnecessary since the discomfort is not great and certainly less than multiple local anaesthetic injections (Fig. 10.1). The tag should be pulled away from the skin and snipped off through the narrowest part of the neck, at the first attempt, just above the junction with the skin. If the tag stump bleeds a small adhesive dressing can be applied to prevent blood staining clothing. Smaller tags rarely bleed; when they do, this usually stops spontane-

Table 10.1 Snip excision of skin tags.

Use sharp fine scissors
No anaesthetic is necessary when snipping off tiny tags
Pull the tag away from the skin using forceps
Snip the tag at its narrowest part
Snip through the neck of the tag
Avoid cutting the tag where it meets the skin — this area is more painful
No haemostatic agent is necessary
Apply a small adhesive dressing to bleeding points
Advise the patient to snip off new tags

Table 10.2 Snip excision of a skin polyp: patient information sheet.

Your skin polyp has been removed. A small wound will remain which will take 1–2 weeks to heal over. The wound should be cleaned daily using cooled boiled water. Remove any debris or crust; apply a thin smear of antiseptic ointment and a small dry dressing. You may shower or bath. After washing, clean the wound as before and apply a clean dressing. If bleeding occurs, apply firm pressure for at least 20 minutes. Once healed the scar may be red and slightly raised. After several months it will settle to a more flesh-coloured flat scar

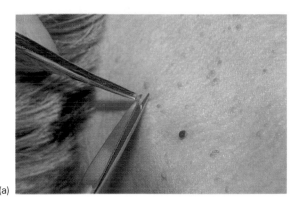

(a)

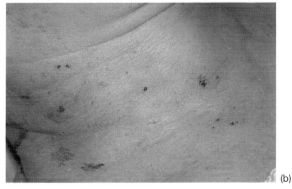

(b)

Fig. 10.1 Snip excision of tiny skin tags. Tiny tags can be snipped off with a pair of sharp scissors without the need for local anaesthetic. The procedure is less painful than a local anaesthetic injection. The tag should be pulled away from the skin and cut at its narrowest point (a). Multiple bleeding points may remain and any that continue to bleed can be covered with a small adhesive plaster (b).

ously within a few minutes. Electrocautery or chemical haemostasis is unnecessary and painful.

New tags will continue to appear and patients can be shown how to snip these off themselves.

Large fibroepithelial polyps

Larger polyps can also be snipped off. Because

large polyps may have a well-developed blood supply, haemostasis is required and thus anaesthetic will be required if cautery is used. The small wound can be left to heal without the need for sutures and this will invariably produce an excellent cosmetic result (Fig. 10.2). Patients can look after the wound themselves very easily (Table 10.2).

Practice points

Histological examination of the multiple tiny tags from typical sites is unnecessary. Diagnosis is straightforward and it seems unlikely that these will ever be confused with a clinically significant alternative diagnosis. Larger polyps may be the

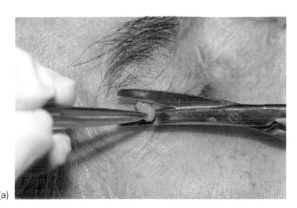

(a)

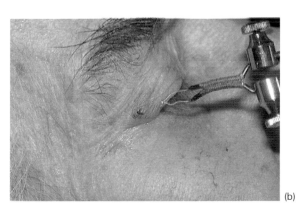

(b)

Fig. 10.2 Snip excision of eyelid skin tag. A larger benign fibroepithelial polyp may require haemostasis, therefore a local anaesthetic is useful. The tag is pulled away from the skin and cut at its narrowest point (a) leaving a small wound

which can be cauterized (b). Electrodesiccation or aluminium chloride haemostasis is equally effective. The resulting wound heals rapidly, producing an excellent cosmetic result.

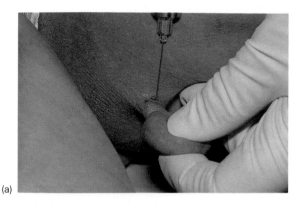
(a)

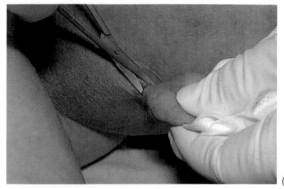
(b)

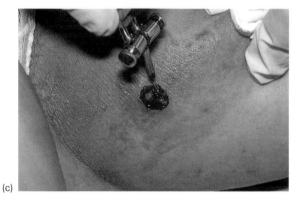
(c)

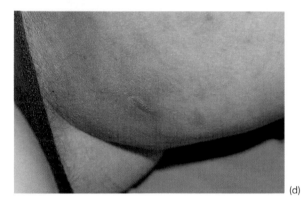
(d)

Fig. 10.3 Snip excision of large soft fibroma. Larger polyps, in this case a soft fibroma, can be excised and sutured but snip excision produces good results. A local anaesthetic is essential (a). Scissors are better than a blade (b) as the crushing effect helps spontaneous haemostasis.

Electrocautery (c), electrodesiccation or a chemical haemostatic agent can be used for haemostasis. The resulting wound will require a dressing (Table 10.2). The cosmetic result at 2 months is satisfactory (d).

Table 10.3 Snip excision of skin tags: patient information sheet.

Your skin tags have been removed. The tiny wounds will take a few days to heal. If they rub on clothing or are sore, apply a thin smear of antiseptic ointment and cover the sore area with a small adhesive dressing. You may shower or bath. If the dressing gets wet remove it, clean the wound and apply a thin smear of antiseptic ointment and a new dressing if required. If new tags appear you can remove these yourself using sterile sharp scissors

result of different pathologies and should be sent for histological examination.

Further reading

Fewkes JL, Change ML & Pollack SV (1992) *Illustrated Atlas of Cutaneous Surgery*. Gower, New York.
Roenigk RK & Roenigk HH (1989) *Dermatologic Surgery: Principles and Practice*. Marcel Dekker, New York.

11: Cautery and electrodesiccation

An electrosurgical unit (Chapter 5) and to a lesser extent an electrocautery machine can be used to treat a variety of benign cutaneous lesions with good cosmetic results.

Equipment

• **Essential:** Electrosurgical unit or electrocautery machine with cold-point tip.

Electrosurgical units vary in their complexity (Chapter 5). A simple unit such as the Birtcher Hyfrecator is adequate for all the procedures described in this book. Several types of cautery tip are available (Fig. 11.1). In dermatological surgery practice the beaded tip is most useful for haemostasis after shave excision (Chapter 12) or curettage (Chapter 9). The cautery blade should not be used as an alternative because this is associated with a small risk of cutting or burning

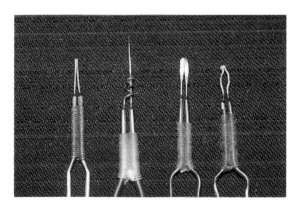

Fig. 11.1 Cautery tips currently available. A beaded tip (far right) is most commonly used. The cautery blade (second right) is used by some to shave off tags or pedunculated lesions but the heat distorts the histological appearance and can only be used effectively if the blade is red hot, i.e. at an unnnecessarily high temperature. Cold-point cautery (second left) can be used to treat spider naevi. The wire tip (far left) has little application in skin surgery.

deeper into the tissue. The cold-point cautery tip is designed to produce a hot sharp needle which can be used to treat spider naevi. Because current will not flow through a single wire, the needle has to be heated, by conduction, via a wire coil. The outer coil does not have to glow red. The correct temperature is reached when the tip is hot enough to scorch a cotton swab. Only 1-second application is required. In the author's experience this method has a slightly greater risk of leaving a scar than electrodesiccation.

Indications

Vascular anomalies such as spider naevi and telangiectasia, xanthelasma and small warts at inaccessible or difficult sites can all be destroyed using cautery or an electrosurgery unit, if treatment is required.

Technique

Spider naevi

Spider naevi can be destroyed using the cold-point tip on an electrocautery machine or electrodesiccated using an electrosurgical unit. When electrocautery is used the power output should be set so that the tip is hot enough to scorch a cotton swab. If local anaesthetic is used it is best to avoid adrenaline as the vasoconstriction will obscure the central feeder vessel. Insert the hot tip into the central feeding blood vessel. Do not press down firmly as this may cause the needle to perforate the full thickness of the skin. Keep the needle in place for less than 2 seconds. The cosmetic result can be reviewed 4–6 weeks later and treatment repeated if necessary.

If an electrosurgical unit is used treatment can usually be tolerated without the need for local

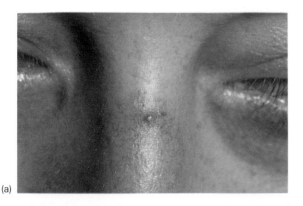
(a)

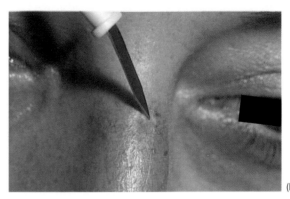
(b)

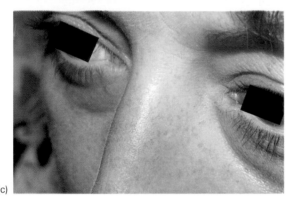
(c)

Fig. 11.2 Electrodesiccation of spider naevus. This spider naevus (a) was treated with a Hyfrecator. Do not take the needle tip off the skin whilst operating the machine as this will cause a tiny spark to flash between the skin and the needle (fulguration — see Chapter 5). This is more painful than electrodesiccation (i.e. when the needle tip is always in contact with the skin) and is less effective. The needle should be sited so that the spider blanches when the tip is pressed on to the skin. Here the site was electrodesiccated for 1 second (b). If the spider does not immediately blanch, the needle can be resited and one more attempt made. In this case the result at 1 month was excellent (c).

anaesthetic (Fig. 11.2). Place the electrosurgical unit tip at the exact centre of the spider naevus and check that it is in the correct position by pressing downwards to ensure that the spider naevus blanches. Remove the pressure but retain contact with the skin. If a Hyfrecator is used, only a 1-second diathermy time is required. Blanching may not be complete initially but do not repeat more than once at each visit because of the risk of scarring (Fig. 11.3). Assess the result after 6 weeks and repeat the treatment if required.

Telangiectasia

Facial telangiectasia, particularly on the nose,

can be destroyed by electrodesiccation using an electrosurgical unit. No local anaesthetic is required. The needle tip is traced along the vessel, which should blanch. The needle tip should remain in contact with the skin at all times so that the vessel is electrodesiccated rather than fulgurized. During fulguration a spark passes between the needle tip and the skin. This is more painful and produces a more superficial skin injury. There is a small risk of linear scarring which is much more obvious on a smooth skin surface.

Xanthelasma

Xanthelasma around the eyelids can be excised

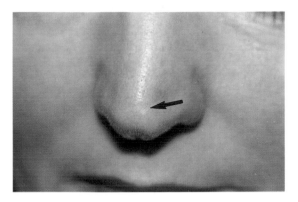

Fig. 11.3 Depressed scar after electrodesiccation of a spider naevus. This spider naevus on the end of the nose was treated on three occasions. Ultimately there was a small depressed scar at the treated site. Always tend to undertreat because of the risk of scarring.

or destroyed in a variety of ways. Electrodesiccation and curettage of the fatty deposits is relatively simple to perform and, unlike some other methods, there is less potential risk of damage to the eye. After local anaesthetic injection the skin over the xanthelasma is disrupted by electrodesiccation and fulguration with the electrosurgical unit (Fig. 11.4). A cautery machine can be used but it is less easy to control the depth of injury. Once the surface has been breached the underlying dermis and its contained fatty deposits can be scraped off using a sharp curette. The area is then fulgurized and electrodesiccated again and left to heal by second intention. Cosmetic results are good and the technique has the advantage over trichloroacetic acid in being predictably effective after one treatment and with less risk of conjunctival injury.

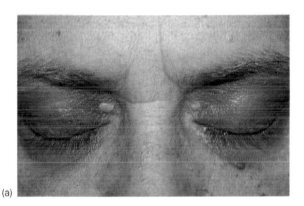

(a)

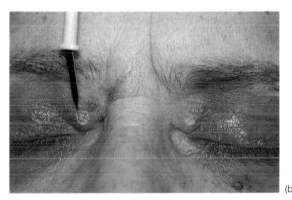

(b)

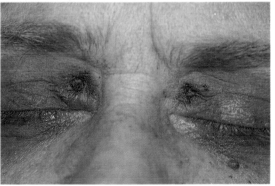

(c)

Fig 11.4 Destruction of xanthelasma using electrodesiccation and curettage. After local anaesthetic injection the epidermis covering the xanthelasma (a) was destroyed (b) by fulguration. The lipid deposits in the underlying dermis can be partially scraped off using a sharp curette (c) and further fulgurized. Complete removal is not usually possible as the yellow material does not scrape off very easily. Any remaining xanthoma deposits disappear spontaneously during the healing process.

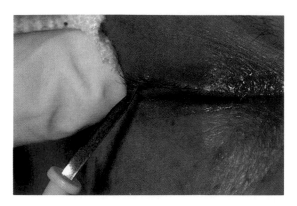

Fig. 11.5 Seborrhoeic wart treatment. Seborrhoeic warts on the eyelid can be treated by desiccation because this treatment can be given very precisely and there is less risk of accidental damage to adjacent important structures, particularly if the lid is pulled away from the eye. Local anaesthetic is usually required. Electrodesiccation softens the wart and the resulting mushy material can be scraped off using a curette if necessary. If there is a risk of conjunctival injury an eye shield can be used (Fig. 4.9).

Small seborrhoeic and plane warts

Smaller plane warts around the eye or on the face can be destroyed using an electrosurgical unit. Fulguration reduces the wart tissue to a mushy consistency which can be curetted off easily. A small part of a more widespread infection of plane wart can sometimes be treated in the hope that this may provoke spontaneous resolution of the remaining warts. Cryotherapy can be used in a similar way. The risk is that treatment will not be successful and a small scar will remain. Plane warts resolve spontaneously in time and if possible they should be left untreated (Table 16.4).

Viral or seborrhoeic warts along the eyelid are difficult to treat with any modality because of the risk of conjunctiva damage. Eversion of the upper lid is a simple technique that enables the lid margin to be treated away from the conjunctiva. Alternatively an eye shield (Fig. 4.9) or eyelid clamp can be used. The latter immobilizes the lid, creates a bloodless field and protects the conjunctiva. Warts on the lid margin can readily be destroyed or softened for curettage using an electrosurgical unit (Fig. 11.5). After local anaesthetic injection the wart is fulgurized or electrodesiccated and when reduced to a soft mushy consistency can be scraped away using a tiny curette. A second cycle of electrodesiccation and curettage may be required.

Practice points

• When treating a spider naevus, warn the patient of the risk of developing a small depressed scar at the treatment site. The risk of this can be minimized by not pressing too hard or treating for longer than 1 second. The lesion should always be treated by electrodesiccation rather than fulguration since the latter is more painful and potentially less effective.

• Try to resist demands to treat spider naevi in children. Spider naevi are common on children's faces. These tend to be smaller than those seen in adults and frequently resolve spontaneously.

• Laser therapy may provide a better and lower-risk alternative for these benign conditions. An argon-pumped tuneable dye laser or flash lamp pump dye laser therapy is probably best for vascular abnormalities on the face. Carbon dioxide laser destruction of xanthelasma is also effective. If a suitable laser is available this could be tried first.

• Since heat is conducted through the skin the discomfort of a hot cautery tip may be felt in the non-anaesthetized adjacent skin.

• Always undertreat because of the risk of scarring. These lesions are all benign and harmless; the only reason for treatment is cosmetic. In these circumstances it is better not to leave a poor cosmetic result.

• Xanthelasma can be destroyed using 95% trichloroacetic acid painted on to the affected area. The technique is not difficult but there is an intrinsic risk of acid getting on to the eye, particularly when the patient starts to produce tears as the acid stings the skin, and repeat treatments are often necessary. Supervised experience needs to be gained before this potentially hazardous procedure is attempted.

• Remember that pigment changes are common after any form of injury in patients with pigmented skin. This includes physical and chemical surgical procedures. Warn the patient of this potential hazard and choose an inconspicuous area as a test area to assess the response before treating other sites.

Further reading

Boughton RS & Spencer SK (1987) Electrosurgical fundamentals. *J Am Acad Dermatol* **16**; 862–867.

Fewkes JL, Cheney ML & Pollack SV (1992) *Illustrated Atlas of Cutaneous Surgery*. JB Lippincott, Philadelphia.

Jackson R (1970) Basic principles of electrosurgery: a review. *Can J Surg* **13**: 354–361.

Pollack SV (1991) *Electrosurgery of the Skin*. Churchill Livingstone, New York.

12: Shave excision

Shave excision is a simple, fast and effective method of removing benign papular naevi. It can also be used as a quick and simple method of obtaining a tissue diagnosis in nodular skin tumours.

Equipment

• **Essential:** local anaesthetic with adrenaline, scalpel blade, haemostatic agent.
• **Optional:** cautery or high-frequency electrosurgical unit.

Indications

Naevi ('moles')

Moles start as flat pigmented junctional naevi, evolve into raised pigmented, compound naevi and mature into flesh-coloured, papular intradermal naevi. These protuberant pigmented and flesh-coloured naevi are a particularly common cosmetic problem on the face. At other sites they tend to catch on combs or rub on clothing. Clinically benign papular naevi are best removed by shave rather than elliptical excision as this frequently creates an excellent cosmetic result, is more easily done and less troublesome for the patient as sutures are not required (Fig. 12.1).

Shave biopsy of skin tumours

If diagnostic biopsy of a tumour is required in order to plan therapy, a simple shave biopsy taken from the surface of the tumour will usually produce sufficient histological material for a pathologist to give a confident diagnosis. An important exception to this is the distinction of keratoacanthoma and squamous cell carcinoma, when a full-thickness biopsy is required. In general, shave biopsy is better for confirming malignancy than supporting a benign diagnosis because of the risk of inadequate sampling.

Technique

Naevi

Inject the local anaesthetic directly into the naevus. This is particularly useful in soft or floppy naevi where it stiffens the tissue and makes it easier to slice off (Fig. 12.2). Hold the blade horizontally flush with the skin when shaving the naevus off. It is easier to mount the blade on a scalpel handle or use a sterile disposable blade, although the blade can be held in the fingers. The shaved naevus must be sent for histological examination.

Haemostasis can be obtained using cautery, electrodesiccation (Chapter 11) or a chemical haemostatic agent (Chapter 5). When using 35% aluminium chloride in isopropyl alcohol, any surface bleeding must first be removed using gauze. The aluminium chloride solution is then applied using a cotton bud dipped in a small quantity of the solution and the tip rolled over the wound surface (Fig. 5.4). Direct pressure may then be required for 1–3 minutes to aid haemostasis. Cautery using a beaded tip is quick and effective and has the advantage of being useful for destroying the edge remnants that commonly remain after shave excision. An electrosurgical machine can be used in a similar way. I do not recommend the use of a blade cautery tip (Fig. 11.1) to slice off the naevus and cauterize bleeding vessels simultaneously, as the cosmetic result achieved is less predictable. A higher heat is required to burn through the tissue, and histological interpretation of the temperature of the specimen will be distorted by heat necrosis artefact. The wound must

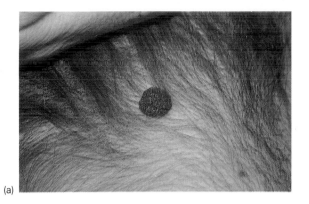

(a)

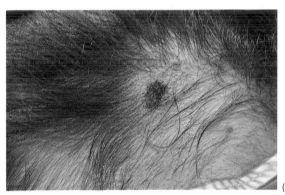

(b)

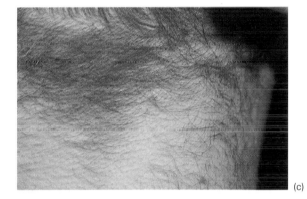

(c)

Fig. 12.1 Shave excision of pigmented naevus. This protuberant warty pigmented naevus (a) was readily shaved off and the wound cauterized (b). At 6 months the cosmetic result was excellent (c). The retention of hair is desirable at hair-bearing sites but may be a problem on other facial naevi. If unwanted hair remains, this can be destroyed by electrolysis.

be kept clean and a small dressing may be required in the first few days (Table 12.1).

The cosmetic results of this technique are good. In approximately 45% of head and neck and 30% of trunk naevi, no visible scar remains. In the remainder the scar is smaller than the original naevus on head, neck and limb sites and a little bigger than the naevus on trunk sites.

Pigmentation remains in approximately 25% of pigmented naevi after shave excision. By contrast, shave excision of non-pigmented naevi rarely, if ever, results in a pigmented scar. Pigmentation may apear at the rim or the centre of the scar (Fig. 12.3). Retained pigment appears to be more common when aluminium chloride is used for haemostasis, by contrast with cautery which may destroy residual naevus cells. Retained pigment does not need to be excised. The original histology will have confirmed the benign nature of the naevus. If the residual pigmentation is excised the pathologist must be given the full

history, since the histological apearances can be difficult to interpret.

Terminal hairs will remain in approximately 20% of cases (Fig. 12.1). The remainder are removed or destroyed by shave excision and cautery. Residual hairs can be destroyed by electrolysis if necessary. Patients should be warned of this possibility and if retained hairs are not acceptable to the patient, the naevus is probably best excised. If the reason for removal is recurrent irritation or frank folliculitis, then formal excision is the treatment of choice.

Shave biopsy of skin tumours

A little anaesthetic is required if cautery is needed for haemostasis (Fig. 12.4). The biopsy is taken by slicing off a segment of the top of the tumour. Bleeding can be stopped using cautery, electrocautery or aluminium chloride. The specimen will be small and fragile so careful transfer to a

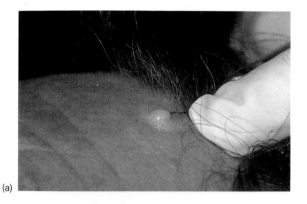
(a)

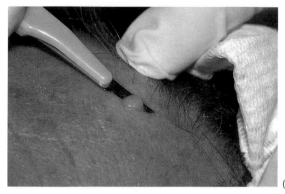
(b)

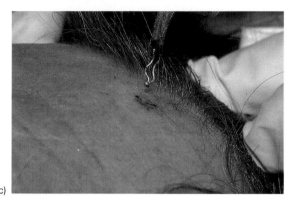
(c)

Fig. 12.2 Shave excision technique. A benign non-pigmented intradermal naevus of the forehead was shaved off. Local anaesthetic was given directly into the mole as this stiffens the tissue and makes it easier to shave off (a). Holding the blade parallel to the skin surface the mole was shaved off (b) flush with the skin, leaving a small circular wound which was cauterized using the beaded tip and an electrocautery machine (c). The resulting wound healed, leaving a scar that was virtually invisible at 3 months.

Table 12.1 Shave excision: patient information.

Your mole has been shaved off. A small wound will remain which will take 1–2 weeks to heal over. The wound should be cleaned daily using cooled boiled water. Remove any debris or crust; apply a thin smear of antiseptic ointment and a small dry dressing. You may shower or bath. After washing, clean the wound as before and apply a clean dressing. If bleeding occurs, apply firm pressure for at least 20 minutes. Once healed, the scar may be red and slightly raised; after several months it will settle to a more flesh-coloured flat scar. Because the technique only removes that part of the mole that protrudes above the skin, brown pigment or hairs, if present initially, may persist in approximately 25% of cases

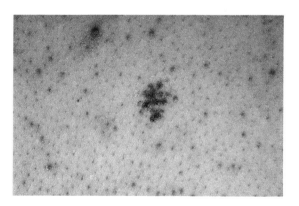

Fig. 12.3 Retained pigment after shave excision of a naevus. Shave excision of pigmented naevi results in pigment retention in approximately 25% of cases. Pigment may be a single central area, scattered or appear around the rim of the shave site.

paper mount is important (Chapter 21). A tumour sometimes bleeds freely when cut and haemostasis can be difficult to achieve. Pressure and aluminium chloride are sometimes more effective than cautery, which tends to burn through the fragile tumour tissue very easily. Do not at-

tempt to take a diagnostic shave biopsy using a curette because the specimen may be fragmented and difficult to interpret.

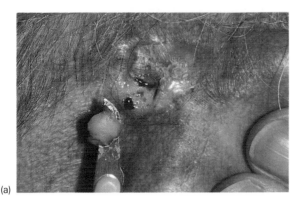

(a)

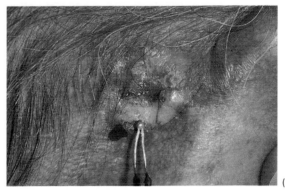

(b)

(c)

Fig. 12.4 Shave biopsy of tumour behind the ear. If a pretreatment biopsy is required, a shave biopsy is frequently adequate. After local anaesthetic injection, a shave biopsy of the thickest area was taken (a). Haemostasis of the shave site was obtained using electrocautery (b), although aluminium chloride would have been equally effective. The specimen was mounted on filter paper and then dropped into formaldehyde (c), so that the specimen did not curl up and distort during fixation.

Table 12.2 Rules of naevus shave excision.

Only shave off unequivocally benign naevi
No scar remains in approximately 45% of head and neck naevi and 30% of other sites
If present, scars are smaller than the original naevus at head, neck and limb sites but slightly bigger on the trunk
Pigment remains in aproximately 25% of originally pigmented naevi
Hair remains in approximately 20% of originally hairy naevi
Shave excision should not be used if residual hair or pigment would be unacceptable to the patient

Practice points

• Remember the fire hazard with alcohol-based skin-cleansing solutions; always use an aqueous skin preparation solution when using cautery or diathermy.

• Shave excision should not be used for biopsy of suspicious pigment naevi. The technique inevitably results in incomplete excision of the naevus, so that the full tumour thickness cannot be measured and there is a debatable increased risk of metastasis after incisional biopsies of malignant melanoma.

• If a flat pigmented naevus would be unacceptable to the patient, excise rather than shave off the naevus (Table 12.2).

Further reading

Hudson-Peacock M, Bishop J & Lawrence CM (1995) Shave excision of benign papular naevocytic naevi *Br J Plast Surg* **48**: 318–322.
Bennet RG (1988) Chapter 14 The skin biopsy. In: *Fundamentals of Cutaneous Surgery*. CV Mosby, St Louis.

13: Elliptical excision, punch biopsy and dog-ear repairs

Elliptical excision and biopsy

This chapter discusses the basic elliptical excision, a more complicated variation called a dog-ear repair, where excision of the lesion and closure of the defect are treated as two separate manoeuvres, and finally, the simple punch biopsy.

Equipment

• **Essential:** local anaesthetic, scalpel and number 15 blade, non-toothed forceps, fine scissors, needle-holder, monofilament suture.
• **Optional:** skin hook, absorbable suture, electro-surgical unit.

Indications

Elliptical excision is essential in the management of suspect moles or naevi but should not be used indiscriminately for the removal of undiagnosed skin lumps and bumps. A variety of benign and malignant skin lesions can be removed, and most incisional skin biopsies are taken using the elliptical excision. The technique is simple but cosmetic results may be poor if the excision is not planned and executed correctly. Moreover, in some situations elliptical excision is inappropriate and produces inferior cosmetic results compared to techniques such as shave excision (Chapter 12), curettage (Chapter 9), punch biopsy (see below) or simply reassurance that surgery is not required. Elliptical excision is indicated when a mole needs to be removed to exclude melanoma (Fig. 13.1). It may also be the most appropriate technique to use when a rash is biopsied, so that the junction between involved and uninvolved skin can be compared. The technique has the advantage that the entire thickness of skin down to fat is excised (Fig. 13.2). Skin tumours can be removed using the technique,

although lesion excision followed by defect repair (see below) is likely to produce superior cosmetic results.

Planning the excision

The ellipse should be designed so that the resulting scar runs parallel to or within an existing skin crease or wrinkle line, provided this does not disturb a critical cosmetic boundary (Fig. 13.3). When skin creases are not visible, for example, in young people or on the trunk or limb, wrinkle lines can be identified by manipulation of the skin (Fig. 13.4) or, on the face, by asking the patient to grimace or smile to accentuate normal skin creases.

The scar must also be as smooth, flat, narrow and short as possible. Scars stretch because insufficient additional support — subcutaneous sutures or tape strips (Chapter 6) — is provided before adequate scar strength develops. Stretching is minimized by placing the wound parallel to the maximum skin tension lines. These lines are generally aligned at right angles to the direction of pull of the underlying muscles (Fig. 8.1).

Technique

Mark the margin to be excised. Choose the optimum direction of closure and design the appropriate ellipse based on these margins. The ellipse length should be approximately three times as long as the width in order for the ellipse angle to be approximately 30°; the angle calcuated should be sufficient to allow skin edges to be pulled together without producing skin buckling. Where there is sufficient skin laxity, this length can be reduced without producing skin buckling. On young or non-wrinkled skin the anticipated ellipse direction is frequently not optimal as it may be difficult to estimate the direction of the maxi-

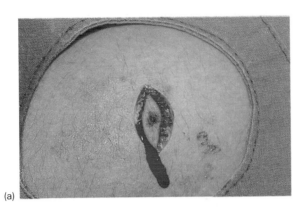

(a)

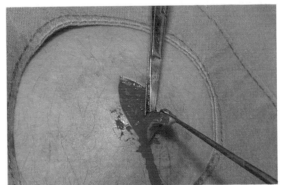

(b)

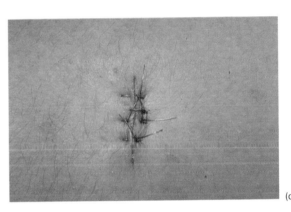

(c)

Fig. 13.1 Elliptical excision of a mole. The mole appeared benign but was reported to be changing in shape and colour. The skin was incised vertically down to fat and the ellipse edges freed from the surrounding skin (a). The remaining fat holding the ellipse in place was cut through using scissors (b). Bleeding points were identified and sealed using a Hyfrecator. The skin edges were undermined to reduce skin tension and subcutaneous sutures used to reduce the risk of the scar stretching or the wound dehiscing when the skin sutures are removed. The sutured edges were everted using vertical mattress sutures to ensure maximal dermis-to-dermis contact (c). A simple dressing was applied.

mum skin tension lines. If there is doubt about the optimum ellipse direction, lesion excision followed by dog-ear repair (see below) may be preferable. The skin should be anaesthetized using the infiltration technique (Chapter 4) so that the lesion and surrounding skin are numb in preparation for undermining. Make each incision as a single continuous sweep rather than a series of small nicks. Ensure that the incision lines meet neatly without crossing over at the tip by starting and finishing each sweep with the blade held vertically (Fig. 13.2c). Incise down to fat. When the ellipse sides and tips are completely separate from the surrounding skin, the ellipse should be sitting on a bed of fat and the fat under the ellipse should be cut through using scissors (Fig. 13.1b), whilst the ellipse is gently pulled away from the skin using a skin hook. If haemostasis is required, use electrosurgical equipment (Chapter 5) or local pressure. The edge of the ellipse must be undermined if there is any tension and this should be done at the appropriate

level (Fig. 8.10) using blunt-tipped scissors or needle-holders. Subcutaneous sutures (Fig. 6.11) should be used to help close the wound if there is any tension. When closing the wound, treat the skin edges gently and do not grip too firmly with forceps. A skin hook is best for this purpose but is potentially hazardous. Ensure the correct suture and technique (Fig. 6.3) are used when closing the wound (Chapter 6). Give patients a wound care advice sheet *before* surgery (Table 13.1) which will also inform the patients that they will have to return for suture removal.

Practice points

• If an elliptical biopsy is done across the boundary between the involved and uninvolved skin, one edge can be marked using typists' correction fluid which should be allowed to dry before the specimen is dropped into formalin. This will remain on the skin surface through histological

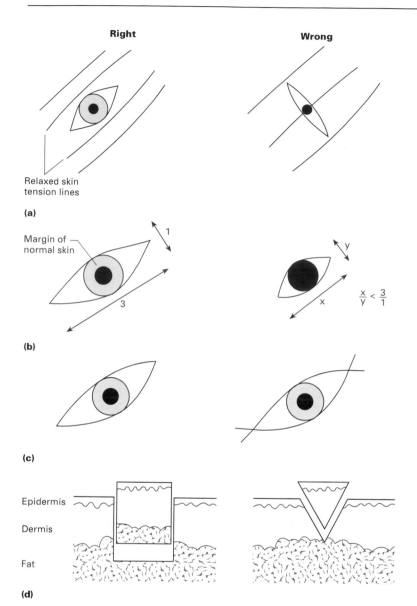

Right

Wrong

Relaxed skin
tension lines

(a)

Margin of
normal skin

1

3

(b)

y

x

$\frac{x}{y} < \frac{3}{1}$

(c)

Epidermis

Dermis

Fat

(d)

Fig. 13.2 Principles of elliptical excision. The ellipse is designed to follow skin-crease lines (a) and should be approximately three times as long as it is wide (b). Ensure that an appropriate margin of normal skin is also excised (b). At the ends of the ellipse hold the blade vertically so that the incision lines do not cross over (c). The blade should be held at 90° to the skin when cutting the ellipse so that the wound has vertical sides down to fat. Do not bevel the blade towards the specimen as this makes the wound more difficult to close and may cut into the dermal component of the lesion (d).

processing and, if the sections are taken longitudinally rather than transversely across the specimen, will appear at one end of the section on the slide as a thin black or opaque line.

• If hair has to be shaved prior to surgery this should be done immediately preoperatively and not the day beforehand, as secondary infection of shaved skin may increase the risk of infection. Hair fragments can be removed using a length of adhesive tape. If the hair is not going to interfere with surgery it does not have to be removed but can be held back with hair grips, tape or gelled into position (see page 90). If shaving is required it is kinder to do it when the area is numb. When suturing in a hair-bearing site choose a suture material that can be easily distinguished from the hair; blue Prolene or Novafil is useful in this respect.

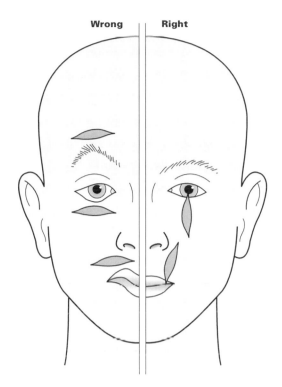

Wrong | **Right**

Fig. 13.3 Planning the ellipse direction. Closure of a large ellipse immediately above the eyebrow may cause unacceptable eyebrow lift, producing a quizzical appearance. Whilst this normally disappears with time, it is best avoided. Excisions of the lower lid should not follow the skin creases if this risks pulling the lower eyelid. This is particularly common in people with weak eyelid tension (Fig. 8.11). Elliptical excisions around the lips should be placed in the radial perioral wrinkle lines to avoid unacceptable elevation of the vermilion border.

• Plan the incision with the patient seated in a relaxed posture. The ellipse shape can be drawn on the skin using a marker pen and Bonney's blue ink (a mixture of crystal violet and brilliant green) or a special skin marker. Do not use ballpoint pen or other felt-tipped pens as the inks may contain carbon particles and there is a small risk of these pigments becoming tattooed into the skin.
• Draping the area with a sterile cotton towel is useful as it prevents hair from getting in the way and is a suitable sterile surface on which to rest instruments. A towel with a central hole can be

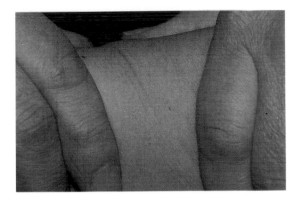

Fig. 13.4 Skin manipulation to identify the direction of relaxed skin tension lines. The skin can be moved between the fingers to identify in which direction the most obvious skin-crease lines run.

Table 13.1 Suture surgery: patient information sheet.

Your wound has been sutured (stitched) and will be sore/tender in 1–2 hours time when the effect of the local anaesthetic wears off. Leave the dressing in place for at least 24 hours or longer if advised to do so. Rest the area. Avoid strenuous exertion for 48 hours. If the wound bleeds, press firmly, continuously and directly over the wound for at least 20 minutes. If bleeding continues despite adequate pressure, seek further medical advice

Keep the area dry for at least 48 hours. Thereafter you should wash, dry and redress the wound. If the wound is painful take paracetamol rather than aspirin since this may provoke bleeding. If you already take aspirin regularly tell your doctor who will advise you about the need to stop therapy

Smoking delays healing. Try to avoid smoking until your stitches are removed

If the wound becomes increasingly painful after 3 or 4 days, contact the doctor

Your stitches will have to be removed 4–12 days after surgery, depending on the site and nature of the operation. Ensure that you are going to be available for stitch removal before agreeing to surgery

Avoid strenuous sport until your stitches are removed and for some time after. Do not go swimming until the wound is fully healed

Once healed the scar may be red and slightly raised; after several months it will settle to a more flesh-coloured flat scar

used, although many patients dislike having their nose and mouth covered. Two smaller towels draped either side of the lesion can be a useful alternative.

• When excising a suspect mole, record the distance between the ellipse margins and the mole (Fig. 13.5), as shown. If the naevus proves to be a malignant melanoma these measurements will enable the surgeon to identify the position of the original naevus and hence re-excise the scar with the appropriate margin.

• Hold the blade at 90° to the skin, not angled inwards. The sides of the excised ellipse and the defect should be vertical (Fig. 13.2). This ensures that the lesion is fully excised and makes the defect easier to close as a full thickness of skin is removed.

• On hair-bearing sites, angle the blade so that it runs parallel to the hair shafts. In this way hair follicles running obliquely through the skin will not be transected, resulting in an unnecessarily wide bald area around the scar.

• If the adjacent skin has to be undermined to allow the edges to be brought together this should be done at the appropriate level (Chapter 8).

• If necessary, close the wound with both absorbable and surface sutures. Subcutaneous sutures will continue to hold the wound edges together after the surface sutures have been removed and will reduce the risk of scar stretching (Chapter 6). When using Vicryl or Dexon (Chapter 6), do not place the suture too high in the skin because of the risk of sutures spitting (Fig. 6.2).

• Orientation of the specimen in the laboratory will be different for an excised lesion compared with an incisional biopsy. Describe clearly on the request form what procedure has been done (Chapter 21).

Excision followed by dog-ear repair

Equipment

• **Essential:** local anaesthetic, scalpel and number 15 blade, non-toothed forceps, curved round-end scissors, needle-holder, skin hook, monofilament and absorbable suture material, electrosurgical unit.

• **Optional:** suction equipment.

Indications

When excising skin tumours it is best to excise the tumour with an adequate margin and then consider the method of repair. Excision will generally leave an oval or circular defect which should first be closed at the centre, possibly creating dog ears or mounds of skin at the corners of the wound which can be removed as necessary (Fig. 13.6). The technique produces a 20% shorter scar than would be created by an equivalent elliptical excision. Furthermore, the possibility of a poorly oriented scar is minimized as the operator is not committed to the direction of the final closure before the defect shape is known and all possible wound-closure directions have been assessed. In most cases the direction of the final scar will be determined by the interaction of the shape excised and the stretching produced by natural skin tension. The usual result is an oval or

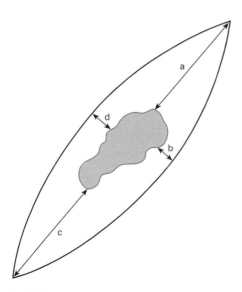

Fig. 13.5 Ellipse measurements prior to suspect mole excision. When excising a suspect naevus, record these measurements so that if the lesion proves to be a melanoma which requires further excision, the operator can identify the site of the original mole and excise the appropriate margin of normal skin.

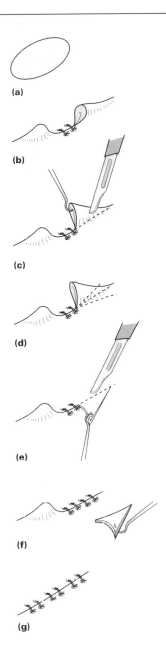

(a)

(b)

(c)

(d)

(e)

(f)

(g)

circular wound, the long axis of which lies parallel to the natural skin tension lines (Fig. 13.7). The skin mobility in different directions is easier to assess once the tumour has been excised and the skin less fixed.

Technique

In a good light, identify the tumour edge and mark the margin of normal skin to be excised around it (Chapter 18). Anaesthetise the skin. Excise the area down to fat or underlying fascia and be prepared to deal with bleeding from small arteries. If bleeding is not excessive, complete the tumour removal stage before attempting to stem the flow of blood from small vessels, as once the tumour is removed a much better view of the area will be gained. Stop bleeding using bipolar or monoterminal diathermy (Chapter 5). Undermine the area around the wound using curved round-ended scissors (e.g. Kilner scissors) and begin to manipulate the skin edges using skin hooks to determine the best possible closure line. Ensure that free skin edges such as the lid or lip are not distorted by these manoeuvres.

Once the best closure line has been established, ensure that the edges are sufficiently mobile to allow the skin edges to be brought together without excessive tension. Place the first few subcutaneous and surface sutures centrally (Chapter 6).

When the central portion of the wound is closed, a dog ear or mound of redundant skin may remain at the tips of the closure. As the skin is elastic and stretches easily, closure of oval wounds does not invariably result in the need for dog-ear repair. In approximately a quarter of wounds closed in this manner there is no need for dog-ear repair at either end. Small dog ears can be

Fig. 13.6 Dog-ear repair. The oval or circular-shaped wound (a) is closed with interrupted subcutaneous and surface sutures as required in the appropriate direction so that the scar will follow the skin creases. (b) The resulting repair has a mound of redundant skin at either end — the dog ears (c). Gentle traction on the dog ear using a skin hook identifies where an incision can be made, joining the wound edge and the point where the skin is flat (c). There are always various direction options at this point: the one that

will result in the most unobtrusive scar, by virtue of following an existing wrinkle line, cosmetic boundary or natural skin crease, should be selected when possible (d). This line is scored with a scalpel and the full thickness of skin cut with scissors. The piece of redundant skin is then draped over the wound edge and the second incision made (e) to complete the removal of the triangle of skin (f). The other end of the wound is treated in the same way (g).

left as these will disappear spontaneously with natural skin tension. Larger ones are repaired as shown (Fig. 13.7). The direction of the dog ear is determined by the operator and, when possible, should be planned to run in an adjacent skin crease or cosmetic boundary. Thus, in many situations this direction is angled away from the wound. The direction of the first incision of the dog-ear repair determines the direction of the scar. The dog-ear length is determined by the amount of tissue that needs to be removed to ensure that the wound lies flat.

Occasionally more than one dog ear is required at one end in order to avoid an important structuresuch as the eye or nose. In these circumstances a so-called W- or M-plasty is created. This is in effect two dog ears taken at an angle of approximately 60° to each other.

Practice points

• This type of surgery should only be attempted when adequate lighting and electrosurgical equipment are available. Suction equipment to remove blood makes the procedure much less stressful for the operator.
• Do not start the procedure if you are not confident about closure. However, if tumour excision results in a larger defect than originally anticipated, remember that some or part of a wound can be left to heal by second intention with good cosmetic results (Chapter 18). It is preferable to have incomplete closure and little tension than massive tension and complete closure since this combination will predispose to ischaemic necrosis followed by wound infection with subsequent

extensive skin loss.
• If the defect is close to the lip, mark the vermilion border before local anaesthetic injection. It is essential when suturing the lip edge that the match is perfect because a stepped vermilion border is difficult to disguise. Skin marker may come off during the procedure. Therefore, mark the vermilion edge adjacent to the excision using a fine suture whilst the skin marker is still visible and the skin is numb.
• Mark important cosmetic boundaries or skin-crease lines before surgery. Once the anaesthetic is in place the subsequent oedema and local anaesthetic-induced temporary paralysis of muscles of facial expression will make it difficult to identify these lines.
• Tissue has to be handled extensively during this procedure and it is important to manipulate the skin edges gently by using a skin hook and not large-toothed forceps to avoid unnecessary damage.

Punch biopsy

Punch biopsies are convenient, quick and produce a relatively small wound which can be allowed to heal by second intention or sutured.

Equipment

• **Essential:** disposable punch biopsy 3 or 4 mm, local anaesthetic.
• **Optional:** non-toothed forceps, sharp iris scissors, needle-holder, monofilament nylon suture material. Electrosurgical unit or aluminium chloride.

Fig. 13.7 (*facing page*) Tumour excision with dog-ear repair. This defect (a) remained after excision of a tumour on the temple (Fig. 8.3). The wound edges were undermined in the avascular plane between the periosteum and the frontalis muscle. The centre of the wound was closed with interrupted surface and subcutaneous sutures (b), thus creating a closure with redundant mounds of skin (dog ears) at either end. The extent of this skin redundancy was identified by lifting the dog ear with a skin hook (c) and one edge of the triangular area of redundant skin was scored

with a blade. This score line was cut with sharp scissors as this gives greater control and hence less risk of producing a ragged skin edge than cutting the full thickness with the blade (d). The triangular piece of skin was draped over the wound to identify the size and shape to be excised (e) and the area excised. The triangular area of skin excised was discarded and the process repeated at the other end, with the incision line designed to run in skin-crease lines where possible and the wound suture (f). The result 2 months later was good (g).

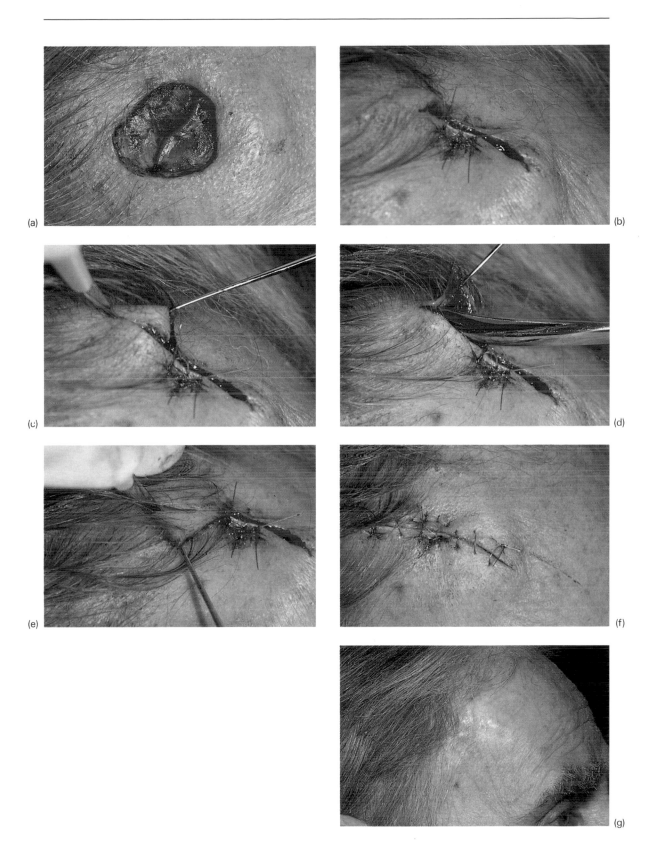

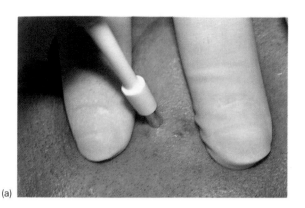

(a)

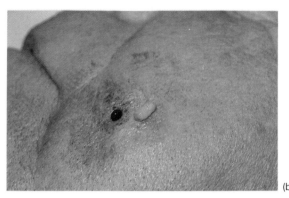

(b)

Fig. 13.8 Punch biopsy of suspect tumour. This nodular subcutaneous tumour was biopsied using the 4-mm punch biopsy. The skin was tensed at right angles to the desired wound closure line (a), the punch inserted and the core of skin removed (b). The biopsy showed it to be a rare Merkel cell tumour of skin.

Indications

Punch biopsy provides a full-thickness excision of the skin down to fat (Fig. 13.8) and can be used to provide confirmation of tumour type when investigating solid tumours but because of the small area sampled cannot, for example, be used to distinguish keratoacanthoma from squamous cell carcinoma or exclude invasion in an actinic keratosis. Punch biopsies are probably most useful in the investigation of inflammatory rashes or skin infiltrates, when multiple punch biopsies may be required. If the pathology is known to be restricted to the epidermis or high dermis, a punch biopsy is unnecessarily deep and provides only a small area of affected skin. In these circumstances a larger but more superficial shave biopsy may provide more appropriate material for the pathologist. A snare biopsy has the advantage that the dermis and follicular epithelium are retained so that re-epithelialization occurs, resulting in a less noticeable scar. Punch biopsies can also be used to excise small lesions such as naevi and the wounds allowed to heal by second intention (Chapter 18). This is a particularly useful technique on the back where smaller scars remain, compared with those created by elliptical excision.

Technique

Disposable punch biopsy blades are widely used and reusable punches are available. Punch sizes range from 2–8 mm although 3- and 4-mm punches are most commonly used. After local anaesthetic injection, drill the punch blade down into fat with gentle downwards pressure. The specimen can then be carefully removed by cutting through the fat at the base with scissors. Punch biopsies produce only very small amounts of tissue albeit a full thickness through to fat. The specimen must be handled carefully so that it is not squashed or the deeper component becomes detached. A punch biopsy may bleed profusely if a small artery is punctured at the base of the wound. The tiny wound makes it difficult to retrieve and diathermy the vessel. If direct sustained pressure does not work, undersewing the punch biopsy using a deep suture is usually effective (see page 23).

Practice points

• Punch biopsy wounds can be sutured or allowed to granulate. The latter takes longer to heal but produces a generally unobtrusive round or oval scar and is appropriate on covered sites.
• The scar of punch biopsy can be minimized by stretching the skin at right angles to the direction in which you want the scar to go. The resulting

wound is narrower in the direction of stretch and hence oval, rather than round, with its long axis parallel to the direction of closure. In effect this usually means that the skin should be stretched at right angles to the wrinkle lines or maximal relaxed skin tension lines whilst the punch is being taken.

• Because only a small area of skin is sampled, care must be taken to biopsy the correct site. In the investigation of rashes, multiple punch biopsies may be required.

• Small punch biopsies may be difficult to orientate in the laboratory. This will limit their value in the evaluation of inflammatory dermatoses but does not usually cause problems for confirmation of a malignant tumour.

Further reading

Borges AF (1982) Dog-ear repair. *Plast Reconstr Surg* **69**: 707–713.

Fewkes JL, Cheney ML & Pollack SV (1992) *Illustrated Atlas of Cutaneous Surgery*. JB Lippincott, Philadelphia.

Hudson Peacock MJ & Lawrence CM (1995) Comparison of wound closure by means of dog-ear repair and elliptical excision. *J Am Acad Dermatol* **32**: 627–630.

Robinson JK (1986) *Fundamentals of Skin Biopsy*. Year Book, Chicago.

Schultz BC & McKinney P (1985) The dermal punch for skin biopsy and small excisions. In: *Office Practice of Skin Surgery*. WB Saunders, Philadelphia, pp. 51–62.

Summers BK & Siegle RJ (1993) Facial cutaneous reconstructive surgery: general aesthetic principles. *J Am Acad Dermatol* **29**: 669–681.

Zachary CB (1991) *Basic Cutaneous Surgery: A Primer in Technique*. Churchill Livingstone, New York.

14: Epidermoid cysts, milia and lipomas

Excision of epidermoid cysts

Epidermoid cysts are sometimes incorrectly called sebaceous cysts. These common cysts are not derived from sebaceous glands. They are lined by a keratinizing epithelium which produces the smelly, cheesy, keratinous contents. Successful removal of an intact epidermoid cyst is a satisfying experience. But scalp cysts can be difficult and time-consuming to remove.

Equipment

• **Essential:** local anaesthetic, number 15 scalpel blade, skin hook, toothed forceps, artery forceps, suture material, needle-holder.
• **Optional:** electrosurgical unit.

Indications

Epidermoid cysts require excision if they are disfiguring or repeatedly infected. Cysts must be distinguished from lipomas, other benign dermal or adnexal tumours. On the scalp, metastatic tumour deposits, cutaneous meningioma and cylindromas may present as nodules. Midline cysts in younger patients may be due to complex developmental abnormalities. Cysts should always be sent for histological examination because basal and squamous cell carcinomas occasionally develop in the cyst wall. Scalp cysts are also produced by pilar (syn. tricholemmal) cysts. These are slightly different to epidermoid cysts in not having a punctum and thus being less likely to become secondarily infected. They are filled with more watery keratinous contents and when the cyst wall bursts there is less of an inflammatory reaction and the retained cyst wall proliferates rather than disintegrates. Occasionally this proliferation can mimic, clinically and histologically, a squamous cell carcinoma. Pilar cysts generally burst more readily than epidermoid cysts.

Infected epidermoid cysts should be *incised* under local anaesthetic, the contents expressed and cultured and an appropriate antibiotic started, based on the assumption that *Staphylococcus aureus* is the infecting organism. Infected cysts are difficult to excise intact because the inflamed tissues are friable. It is best to let the inflammation settle and then excise the cyst.

Cysts may also become inflamed because the cyst wall ruptures after being squeezed. The released keratin causes a foreign-body giant-cell reaction in the surrounding tissues. Such cysts are tender but there is less surrounding inflammation and what inflammation there is lasts longer compared to an infected cyst. Inflamed cysts are best treated by the injection of triamcinolone (10 mg/ml, 1–2 ml) into the cyst. This usually results in the spontaneous resolution of the entire cyst. If the nodule remains it can be removed when all the inflammation has settled.

Technique

Mobile cysts

The method adopted depends on how mobile the cyst is. Freely mobile cysts can be removed intact by shelling out the cyst. It is important to find the correct tissue plane which is immediately next to the cyst wall. At this level the cyst wall is smooth and easily separates from the surrounding tissue. It is however very easy to puncture the fragile cyst wall and the tissues must be handled gently. Removal of the complete cyst reduces the risk of leaving a fragment of cyst wall behind, which may result in recurrence (Fig. 14.1). It is important to excise the punctum, if present, within a small ellipse of skin. The cyst can be gripped

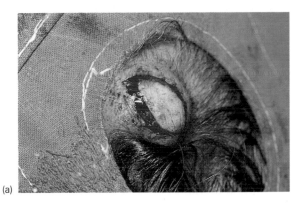
(a)

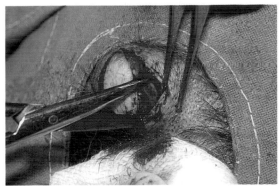
(b)

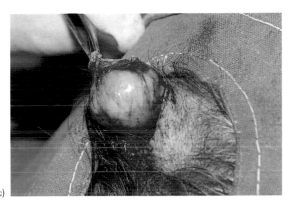
(c)

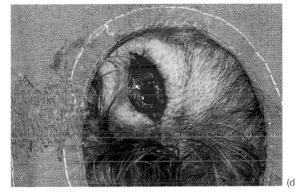
(d)

Fig. 14.1 Excision of intact epidermoid cyst. Inject local anaesthetic around but not into the cyst. On the scalp, hold the blade parallel to the hair shafts and excise an ellipse of skin to include the punctum if present (a). Blunt-dissect around the cyst to free it (b). Try not to burst the cyst, as remaining wall fragments may result in a recurrence. The ellipse of skin can be used to grasp the cyst but will have to be treated gently or it may be pulled off the cyst wall (c). Any remaining dead space (d) must be obliterated with subcutaneous sutures or a pressure bandage. Redundant skin need not be excised, as it will shrink back to its correct size in time.

using this ellipse rather than the fragile cyst wall.

Alternatively a mobile cyst can be punctured, the contents expressed and the furthermost portion of the cyst inner wall grasped with the tip of a pair of artery forceps, pulled inside out through the skin wound and ultimately pulled out of the wound. Care has to be taken to ensure that the complete cyst wall is removed as this may fragment if pulled too hard.

If the cyst is very large and excision would result in a long scar, the cyst size can be first reduced by expressing the cyst content through a skin punch excision. This should include any punctum if present. The remaining cyst wall can then be removed through a smaller incision. If there is any inflammation present this should be allowed to settle and the remaining cyst wall removed through a smaller wound approximately 6 weeks later (Fig. 14.2).

Immobile cysts

Cysts that have been repeatedly squeezed or infected are usually stuck to the surrounding tissue and overlying skin. These are surrounded by extensive scar tissue and cannot be removed very easily. It is usually necessary to excise the surrounding fibrotic tissue and overlying skin. This requires extensive, time-consuming, blunt dissection through the surrounding dermal tissues.

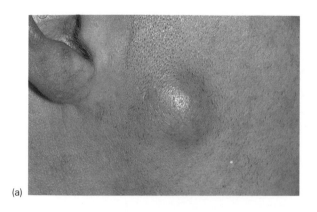
(a)

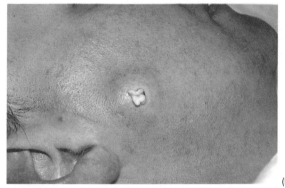
(b)

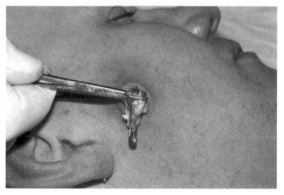
(c)

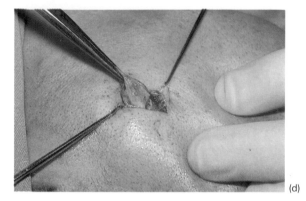
(d)

Fig. 14.2 Removal of large cyst through smaller wound. Routine removal of large cysts will inevitably result in large scars (a). Alternatively, a 3–4-mm punch biopsy hole can be made through the skin over the cyst, to include the cyst punctum if present, and the contents expressed (b). The cyst size is thus greatly decreased and in non-inflamed cysts the collapsed cyst wall may be removed through the punch excision by grasping the inside of the cyst using a pair of artery forceps (c). Because the cyst wall tears easily, especially if the tissues are inflamed, complete removal can be difficult, as in this case. Thus, here the cyst contents were expressed and only part of the cyst removed. The punch biopsy site was left to heal without sutures and 6 weeks later the inflammation had subsided and the punch excision site had healed. The remaining cyst was then removed through a smaller wound (d).

Practice points

• Scalp surgery can be difficult. The wound is obscured by hair and bleeding is profuse. Thus, sufficient time, an assistant and adequate equipment are essential. Shave enough hair to ensure that the operation site can be seen clearly. Hold surrounding hair out of the way with tape or lubricating jelly used as a hair gel. In the scalp make the incision parallel to the hair shafts. This avoids damaging too many follicles and thus results in a narrower bald area adjacent to the scar.

Do not delegate the task to an inexperienced junior on the basis that 'it is just a cyst'.
• The scalp bleeds profusely and a lot of blood may run down on to the back of the patient's neck. Rest the patient's head on a thick towel or absorbent pad and drape the neckline with polythene to prevent blood soiling clothing.
• It is sometimes difficult to distinguish dark scalp hair from suture material. Use a bright blue suture material like Prolene or Novafil (Chapter 6) to overcome this problem.
• A long needle is needed to pass through the

entire thickness of the scalp. This also has to be robust so that it does not bend or break when pushed through the scalp (e.g. number 3 suture with 22-mm needle). If the needle starts to bend, consider replacing it before it breaks because a lot of time can be wasted searching for a broken needle in the wound.

Excision of lipomas

A lipoma can be excised simply by making an incision over the centre of the nodule down to fat and removing the lipoma. In patients with multiple lipomas this results in multiple scars. Scar size can be kept to a minimum by breaking up the lipoma prior to excision and expressing the fragments through a smaller wound.

Equipment

• **Essential:** local anaesthetic, number 15 scalpel blade, skin hook, toothed forceps, artery forceps, suture material, needle-holder.
• **Optional:** electrosurgical unit.

Indications

Lipomas may have to be removed because they are painful or disfiguring. Lipomas have usually been present for several years, slowly increasing in size. Rapidly enlarging subcutaneous or dermal nodules may be produced by primary or secondary tumours or occasionally inflammatory nodules. Angiolipomas are sometimes spontaneously painful. Lipomas may be distinguished from cysts by their smooth lobulated surface and the absence of a punctum.

Technique

Removal of a lipoma can be done very simply. A single incision is made over the centre of the nodule, the lipoma removed, bleeding points identified and diathermied and the skin edges sutured.

If a smaller scar is desirable, and this is particularly so in patients with multiple lipomas, large lipomas can be removed through a small scar (Fig. 14.3). A 4–6-mm punch biopsy or linear incision can be made over the centre of the lipoma. The lipoma is then broken up using blunt dissection with round-end scissors or artery forceps and the fragments squeezed out through the wound. Considerable pressure is required initially but once the first few fragments have been expressed the rest will come out more easily. Blunt dissection must be done carefully so that no vital structures are damaged. This is achieved by gripping the lipoma between the finger and thumb of one hand and blunt-dissecting with the other. In this way the lipoma can be held away from underlying structures and the depth of dissection gauged by the fingers holding the lipoma. Some lipomas are very fibrous and cannot be fragmented. If this happens, or there is significant bleeding into the dead space, the incision may have to be extended before the lipoma can be removed.

Practice points

• After removal of the lipoma there may be some skin laxity. Rather than excise the apparently excess skin, the edges can be sutured. Any dead space should be obliterated with a pressure bandage or subcutaneous suture. The skin laxity will disappear spontaneously once the distension has gone.
• Lipomas may recur if lipoma cells remain, so attempt to remove the entire lesion.

Milia removal

Milia are tiny keratin-filled, epithelial-lined cysts, common on the face. Unlike the closed comedones that occur in acne, they are not connected to the skin surface so a small skin incision has to be made before they can be removed.

Equipment

• **Essential:** Sterile venesection needle (21- or 19-gauge).
• **Optional:** Fine-toothed forceps.

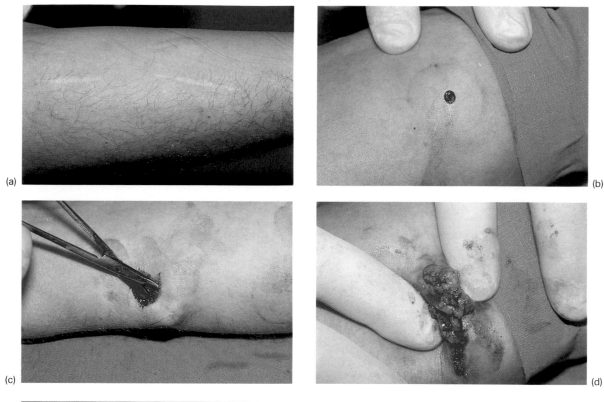

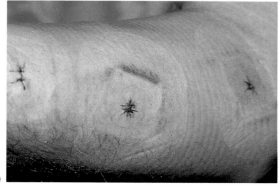

Fig. 14.3 Lipoma removal. Excision of multiple lipomas results in multiple scars, as here (a). Soft mobile lipomas can be expressed through tiny excisions. A 4-mm punch biopsy hole was made through the skin over the centre of the lipoma (b). The lipoma can be broken up by blunt dissection (c), using artery forceps, and the fragments squeezed out through the 4-mm hole (d). The entire lipoma should be removed to guard against the possibility of recurrence. Bruising is inevitable around the surgery site; a firm pressure bandage must be used to limit postoperative haemorrhage (e).

Indications

Milia appear and resolve spontaneously. There is no real need to remove these, although patients frequently find them cosmetically troublesome.

Technique

No anaesthetic is required. The skin over the milium is pierced by the tip of the needle and then the skin incised using the cutting edge of the bevelled tip of a venesection needle (Fig. 14.4). The milium can then be lifted out on the tip of the needle or gently squeezed out through the incision, using fine-tipped forceps or a comedone expressor.

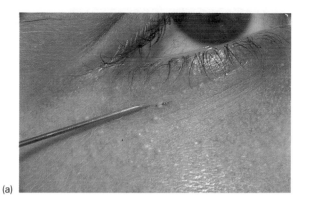
(a)

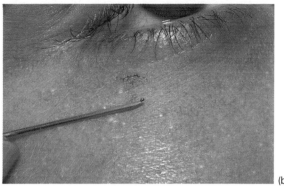
(b)

Fig. 14.4 Milia removal. Milia are common on the cheeks of young adults. Use a venesection needle with the cutting edge held perpendicular to the skin surface to cut through the skin over the milia. First prick the needle into the skin (a) and cut through the skin from beneath upwards. The cyst can be hooked out (b) on the needle or squeezed out using forceps.

Practice point

• Correct technique takes practice and it is too time-consuming to remove all the milia in a patient. The technique can be demonstrated to the patient or companion who can complete the task.

Further reading

Epstein E & Epstein E Jr (eds) (1987) *Skin Surgery.* WB Saunders, Philadelphia.

Roenigk HR & Roenigk RK (eds) (1989) *Dermatologic Surgery: Principles and Practice.* Marcel Dekker, New York.

15: Nail avulsion and ingrown toenail

Nail avulsion

Equipment

• **Essential:** plain local anaesthetic, fine scissors, robust forceps (e.g. Spencer Wells 6-in), tourniquet.
• **Optional:** nail elevator (e.g. Francis elevator or small nail elevator).

Indications

Nail removal is required prior to biopsy of suspected tumours of the nail bed or matrix. Stubborn toenail, but not fingernail, fungal infections sometimes only respond to a combination of nail avulsion and oral antifungal therapies. Occasionally trauma may so damage the nail plate that avulsion of the nail and allowing a new one to regrow is a reasonable option.

Avulsion alone is not a useful treatment for ingrown toenails. This procedure results in temporary relief but is associated with a high recurrence rate if no further therapy is offered.

Technique

A ring block (Fig. 4.7) of the affected digit using plain lignocaine is the most effective way of producing digit anaesthesia and also removes the pain of the tourniquet, which should be applied immediately before surgery (Fig. 15.1). On the finger this can be done by the patient wearing a snug-fitting sterile rubber glove. The affected glove fingertip end is cut and the rubber rolled back down the finger, producing a tight tourniquet at the base of the finger. The sterile glove obviates the need to cover the rest of the hand in a sterile drape and the process of rolling the rubber back down the finger empties the finger of

blood, thus preventing venous engorgement producing bleeding when the finger is first incised. A less elegant method for both fingers or toes is simply to wind a sterile piece of Paul's tubing around the finger and hold it in place using an artery forceps. The rubber-band technique can also be adapted to produce an exsanguinating tourniquet if applied using Esmarch's technique (Fig. 15.1).

The junction between the nail plate and posterior and lateral nail folds is separated using a nail elevator (Fig. 15.2). A pair of sharp scissors can be used for this purpose but may potentially puncture the nail fold. The connection between the nail plate and nail bed is breached distally by blunt dissection using the nail elevator. The gap under the nail is enlarged until the nail plate can be grasped along its full length with a large needle-holder. The nail is then rolled off the nail bed by gripping the loose edge of the nail and rotating the forceps towards the other lateral nail fold. It is important to ensure that the entire nail, including the nail horns, is removed. If the nail splits whilst being rolled off the nail bed, the process will have to be repeated until the entire nail is removed.

Practice points

• Some people find nail surgery gruesome to watch. Ask these individuals to leave the room in case they faint.
• On fingers limit the volume of lignocaine injected to approximately 3–4 ml depending on the size of the digit because of the risk of blocking blood flow by injecting large volumes into a small space. Never inject more anaesthetic after the tourniquet has been applied for the same reason.
• The time of tourniquet application and removal should be recorded in the notes. Digit

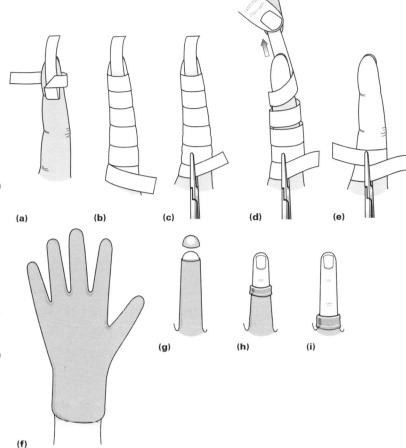

Fig. 15.1 Tourniquet application. An exsanguinating tourniquet can be created using an Esmarch bandage. The aim is to squeeze blood out of the digit by winding the tourniquet round it starting at the tip, where a loop is created with the first turn (a), and finishing at the base (b), where the tourniquet is clamped (c). When the tourniquet has been clamped, the loop is tugged to release the distal end of the tourniquet and reveal the nail. Alternatively, the patient puts on a sterile glove one size too small (f); the fingertip is cut off (g); the finger end is rolled back, ensuring this is as broad as possible (h). This squeezes out the blood as it is rolled back and then acts as a tourniquet when it reaches the base of the finger (i).

(a) (b) (c) (d) (e)

(f) (g) (h) (i)

tourniquets should only be left on for approximately 20 minutes and this is particularly important in patients with an impaired limb blood supply, such as diabetics. Many authors suggest that tourniquets can be left on for up to 60 minutes in healthy adults. The two tissues at risk when a tourniquet is used are nerve and muscle and it is the risk of direct nerve damage, rather than muscle necrosis, which limits the tourniquet time on the finger. Very high local pressures can be created when a rubber-band tourniquet is applied rather than a pneumatic cuff because the band may be very narrow and there is no way of monitoring the pressure achieved, which may be far in excess of that required to stop blood flow.

The rubber band used should therefore be as broad as possible (Fig. 15.2) and the time kept to the minimum. If the operation is longer than anticipated, the tourniquet can always be temporarily removed and reapplied.

• Oedema frequently occurs postoperatively, especially if a tourniquet has been used, thus a tight or circular bandage should always be avoided.

• Once the procedure is finished the dressing can be applied. A greasy ointment covered by paraffin gauze is useful as this aids dressing removal later. The tourniquet is removed and the toe checked to ensure that the blood flow has been re-established. A larger dressing is then applied using a crêpe bandage wound around the toe. It is

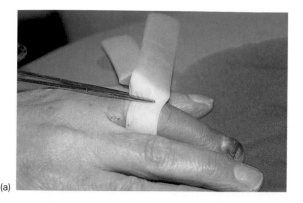
(a)

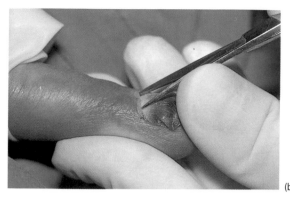
(b)

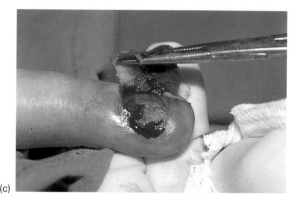
(c)

Fig. 15.2 Nail avulsion. The patient had a solitary dystrophic fingernail. After ring block a wide tourniquet was applied (a). The connection between the nail plate and the posterior nail fold and end of the finger were separated using fine scissors (b). Blunt dissection using a nail elevator is an alternative but may be difficult to use in non-inflamed tissue which does not separate so easily. When the nail is freed sufficiently for it to be gasped by the needle-holder, the nail plate is gripped along its full length and rolled off the nail bed (c). The exposed nail bed appeared normal.

not necessary to anchor this to the foot or ankle but the bandage should include pleats to allow for expansion and prevent the dressing from constricting the toe. This can be held in place with two pieces of adhesive tape, which should not be wound around the toe for the same reason.
• The dressing should be soaked off after 48 hours. The nail will take 8–9 months to regrow. The ventral nail or nail bed will harden up before the nail plate completely regrows and a dressing will be unnecessary after approximately 6 weeks.
• Non-surgical removal of dystrophic fungal-infected nails using 40% urea ointment is an alternative if surgery is impossible.

Treatment of ingrown toenail

Equipment

• **Essential:** plain local anaesthetic, fine scissors, robust forceps, liquid phenol BP, nail splitter

(e.g. Thwaites nail nipper), tourniquet, nail elevator.

Indications

Ingrown toenails are caused by incorrect nail cutting, which results in a tiny spicule of nail at the free edge growing into the lateral nail fold, producing inflammation and ultimately perforation of the lateral nail-groove epithelium. In the acute phase the aim is to relieve discomfort. Once inflammation has settled the aim is to prevent recurrence.

Technique

Acute phase

In the acute inflammatory phase simple antiseptics, treatment of secondary infection and anti-inflammatory therapy are usually all that is required. It is also sometimes possible to lift the ingrowing corner portions of the nails clear of the lateral nail fold by twisting a small pledget of cotton wool under the nail in the lateral nail fold. Once all the inflammation has settled it is then necessary to perform surgery that will prevent the condition from recurring. Lateral matrixectomy involves removal of the side of the nail and destruction or removal of the nail matrix. This produces a narrow but cosmetically acceptable nail. The matrix is most effectively and simply destroyed using liquid phenol.

Prevention of recurrence

The toe is anaesthetized and a tourniquet applied. A bloodless field is important when phenol is used because blood inactivates phenol and thus any venous oozing may prevent the phenol from destroying the nail matrix; an exsanguinating Esmarch tourniquet is thus preferred. The nail plate is blunt-dissected from the lateral and posterior nail folds and from the nail bed using a nail elevator. An approximately 4 mm wide portion of the nail plate is then cut completely through from distal margin to matrix using the nail splitter (Fig. 15.3). A scalpel should not be used as it may slip or break on a hard toenail. The fragment of nail is then grasped using a robust needle-holder or forceps and twisted off so that the entire length of nail, including the lateral horn, is removed. Debris and granulation tissue in the lateral nail fold can be removed with a curette. The nail matrix is then destroyed using 90% phenol BP. This should be done using an orange stick and a small piece of cotton wool. The tip is dipped in the phenol and this is pushed firmly into the nail matrix. In this position the cotton bud should be rotated towards the centre of the nail to pull any debris away from the lateral horn because tissue fragments wedged in the matrix horn may shield the horn matrix from the effect of the phenol. After a minute the applicator should be removed and replaced with a fresh phenol-dipped applicator held in place for a further minute. Take particular care to ensure that the horn or lateral tip of the nail matrix receives

sufficient treatment because most of the 1–2% of cases that recur arise from this area.

Practice points

• Prevention is better than cure. Show patients how to cut their toenails properly so that the corners of the nails protrude beyond the lateral nail folds (Fig. 15.4).
• In the acute phase, consider referral to a qualified chiropodist as chiprodists are frequently able to deal with the problem very effectively.
• The nail matrix can also be excised. Surgical matrixectomy takes longer and has to be done properly to avoid the risk of incomplete removal of the matrix horns.
• Phenol is caustic and great care must be taken not to allow drips to fall on the patient's normal skin. To be fully effective, a bloodless field is essential, otherwise this will effectively neutralize the phenol before it has an effect on the matrix. The exsanguinating tourniquet technique is required (Fig. 15.1). Before phenol application, remove any blood using a dry cotton-tip applicator. Remember to discard immediately all swabs or cotton buds that have been in contact with phenol so that they cannot be mistakenly used to clean the wound.
• The toe should be tipped slightly towards the affected side so that phenol does not track centrally towards the normal matrix. There is no need to neutralize the phenol after application but any residual phenol must be wiped off so that the surrounding skin is not damaged.
• Use wooden orange-stick applicators and not plastic cotton buds when handling phenol as this may melt the plastic.
• Pincer nails caused by an inherent transverse over-curvature of the nail are another cause of ingrown toenails. Both lateral nail-plate edges dig into the nail bed rather than the lateral nail fold. Although more obvious on the big toe, it is also present on all toes. The same method of treatment can be employed but both edges have to be removed, which leaves a much narrower nail.
• Phenol application can be used to destroy the

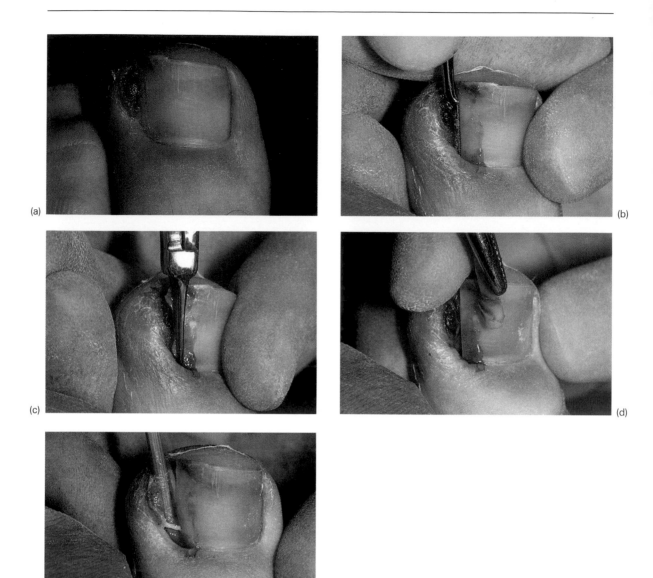

Fig. 15.3 Phenol matrixectomy of an ingrown toenail. After local anaesthesia this typical ingrown toenail (a) was treated by phenol ablation of part of the nail matrix. The junction between the lateral and posterior nail folds was blunt-dissected using a Francis nail elevator (b). When the side of the nail was free, approximately 4 mm of nail was snipped off using the Thwaites nail splitter or nipper (c). This has a lower anvil-like surface and an upper cutting blade. The piece of nail was grasped with robust needle-holders and pulled free of the nail bed (d). The removed portion consisted of the complete length of nail with a ragged lateral edge. In this case there was no true spicule of nail. The wound was dried using a cotton bud and then liquid phenol applied using an orange stick lightly wrapped in cotton wool. Before use, a small quantity of phenol should be poured into a steel galley pot as phenol melts plastic. The tip of the orange stick was placed in the lateral nail fold and nail matrix (e) and rotated towards the centre of the nail to prevent tissue fragments from masking the nail matrix from the effect of the phenol. Two 1-minute phenol applications were used. A dressing was applied. (This patient was treated by the students and staff of Durham School of Podiatric Medicine, New College, Durham.)

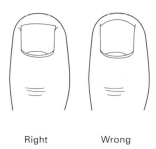

Right   Wrong

Fig. 15.4 Correct nail-cutting technique. Cut the nail so that the corners of the nail protrude beyond the lateral nail folds (a) and not back into the lateral nail folds (b).

entire nail. The technique is similar to that described above, except that after complete nail removal, three 1-minute phenol application times are used, rolling the applicators from horn to horn of the matrix.

Further Reading

Baran R & Dawber RPR (eds) (1994) *Diseases of the Nails and their Management*, 2nd edn. Blackwell Scientific, Oxford.

Butterworth R & Dockery GL (1992) *A Colour Atlas and Text of Forefoot Surgery*. Wolfe, London.

Lorimer DL (ed.) (1993) *Neale's Common Foot Disorders: Diagnosis and Management. A General Clinical Guide*, 4th edn. Churchill Livingstone, Edinburgh.

Wallace WA, Milne DD & Andrew T (1979) Gutter treatment for ingrowing toe nails. *Br Med J* **2**: 168–171.

16: Treatment of viral warts

Types of viral wart

There are currently 55 recognized human papillomavirus (HPV) types. Clinical appearance is determined by both HPV type and wart site (Table 16.1). Left to grow unhindered, the common wart is a filiform exophytic papule (Fig. 16.1, Fig. 17.2). On the fingers the filiform extensions are worn away, leaving the warty papule. On the sole the wart is pushed into the skin to form the characteristic plantar wart or verruca. When multiple, confluent tiny warts are present on the sole, a so-called mosaic wart is produced. These are much more difficult to treat than

Table 16.1 Human papillomavirus (HPV) types associated with clinical lesions.

Clinical appearance	HPV types
Common warts	1,2,4,7
Plane (flat) warts	2,3,10,26–29
Meat, fish, poultry-handlers' warts	2,7
Genital warts	6,11,16,18,30–32,42–44,51–55
Bowenoid papulosis	16,18,31,32,34,39,42,48,51–54
Cervical dysplasia	16,18,31,32,35,42,51–54
Cervical carcinoma	16,18,31,32,33,35,39,42,51–54

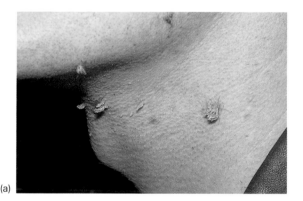

(a)

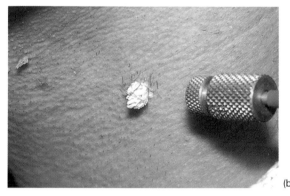

(b)

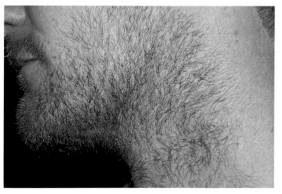

(c)

Fig 16.1 Cryotherapy of warts on face. These filiform warts on the beard area (a) will spread around the face very quickly if the patient continues to shave. Cryotherapy is relatively effective when the wart is as exophytic as this (b). The patient was asked to stop shaving and the warts treated on three occasions, with a good outcome 2 months later (c). Cryotherapy can cause permanent scarring alopecia if long freeze times are used.

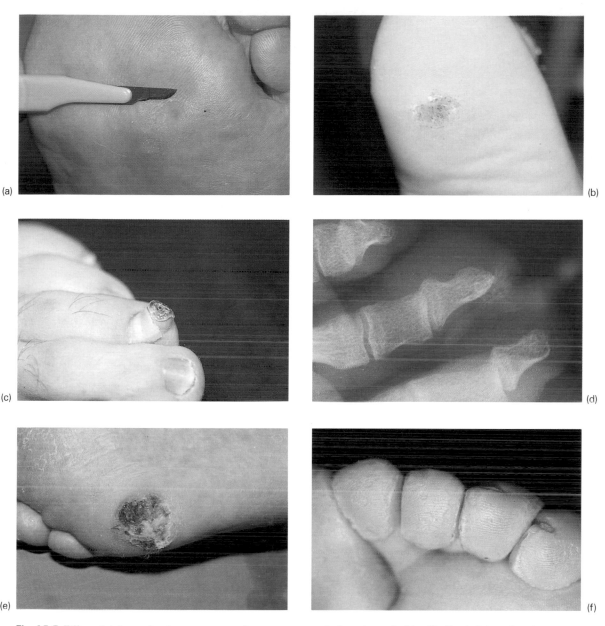

Fig. 16.2 Differential diagnosis of common wart. A corn usually arises over the head of the tarsal bones. It can be distinguished from a wart on paring, when the corn continues to show the clear yellow waxy keratin (a), whereas the small thrombosed or bleeding blood vessels appear in the wart (b). Subungual exostosis (c) is occasionally confused with periungual warts. The X-ray appearance is characteristic (d). Squamous cell carcinomas (carcinoma cuniculatum) must be identified by their irregular edge, steadily increasing size and nodularity (e). Pitted keratolysis is caused by a *Corynebacterium* infection of the keratin and results in the characteristic pitted appearance and very smelly feet (f). This can be treated with topical antibiotics to destroy the bacteria or 2% formaldehyde soaks to reduce sweating and the conditions in which the bacteria thrive.

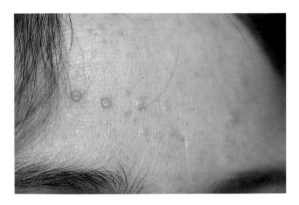

Fig. 16.3 Molluscum contagiosum of the forehead. Note the characteristic umbilicated centre.

simple plantar warts. Other foot dermatoses must not be confused with plantar warts (Fig. 16.2).

Molluscum contagiosum is produced by a poxvirus but is considered in this section as some treatment options are the same as for HPV infections. This virus has an incubation period of between 15 and 50 days. The umbilicated papules are up to 10 mm in diameter (Fig. 16.3). Lesions may occur at injury sites and are common in atopic eczema sufferers. Eczema may occur around mollusca in 10% of patients who otherwise do not suffer from eczema.

Treatment options

No therapy

Five per cent of 16-year-old British schoolchildren have common warts. Approximately two-thirds of common warts disappear spontaneously within 2 years. Resolution is not influenced by the patient's age or the number of warts. Plane warts sometimes only become apparent when they begin to resolve spontaneously. All these types of wart can reasonably be left untreated. By contrast, genital warts should always be treated because they are highly infective and probably cause female genital tract cancers (Table 16.1). Adults with genital warts must always be examined for other sexually transmitted disease, so referral to a genitourinary medicine department

is more useful than referral to a dermatologist. Genital warts in children may be a sign of sexual abuse.

Molluscum contagiosum infection usually lasts 6–9 months. Spontaneous remission is preceded by inflammation, suppuration and crusting of the papule. On resolution a small scar may be apparent, but this becomes invisible in time.

Medical therapies

Salicylic acid and lactic acid therapy

These keratolytic agents work by encouraging shedding of the infected keratinocytes. There is little to choose between the various commercial preparations. The single most important factor in treatment success is patient motivation and understanding of the principles of treatment (Table 16.2). The agents that dry leaving an elastic film on the skin are easier to use as no dressing is required and there is less irritation on the skin. When used correctly, the cure rate of 70% is identical to that achieved using liquid nitrogen. Combining keratolytic therapy and liquid nitrogen is more effective than either therapy alone. Salicylic acid remedies are not advised for the treatment of warts on the face because of the risk of the solution getting into the eye.

Formaldehyde soaks

Mosaic warts are difficult to treat and at best cure rates of 50% are all that may be expected. Because

Table 16.2 Treatment using salicylic acid/lactic acid preparations.

Treat the wart once a day. Do not treat if the wart is painful
Rub away the wart surface using an emery board or hard-skin scraper
Soak the foot for 10 minutes in warm water. Keep your towel separate from others
Apply 1–2 drops of the salicylic acid solution using the applicator so that the wart surface is just covered
Consult your doctor to confirm that the wart has gone before stopping treatment
If the wart becomes painful, see your doctor

Table 16.3 Regimen for formaldehyde soaks.

Treat the wart daily. Do not treat if the wart is painful

Protect the normal skin with a liberal application of Vaseline before formaldehyde application

Dip the affected area in the 12% formaldehyde solution for 10 minutes. Excess formaldehyde can be poured back into the bottle and reused

Wash the foot with soap and water. Keep your towel separate from others

Do not cover the treated area

Pare the warts weekly as shown

wide areas are affected, locally destructive therapies are not successful. The author uses 12% formaldehyde solution soaks applied to the skin for 10 minutes each day (Table 16.3). The surrounding normal skin must be protected with Vaseline (Fig. 16.4). The warts should be pared weekly using an emery board, razor or hard-skin scraper, depending on the patient's dexterity and eyesight. As with all wart therapies, treatment should be missed if the wart becomes painful. Clearance takes at least 3 months.

Podophyllin

This is useful for the treatment of friable genital warts but has little effect on hard genital warts. Applications of the solutions discussed here should be applied by trained staff and not by the patient. Start using 15% podophyllin paint, compound BP, which is applied using a cotton-wool bud (Fig. 16.5). The area is dusted with talcum powder immediately after to help absorb any excess. The patient is advised to wash off the solution after 6–8 hours or earlier if painful. Repeat applications can be applied weekly. Podophyllin is hazardous in very young children or pregnant women because of a potential neurotoxic effect and has once been reported to produce stillbirth. Podophyllin paint (15%) may be used on stubborn plantar warts but is no more effective than salicylic acid preparations (Table 16.4).

Others

Plane warts are difficult to eradicate and weak salicylic acid or retinoic acid applications are advocated (Table 16.4).

Cryotherapy

Freezing does not kill wart viruses. Cryotherapy works by destroying the tissue in which the virus lives and possibly by enhancing the immune response to the virus. The wart and a small rim of apparently normal tissue must be frozen;

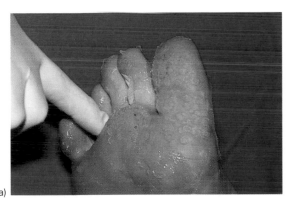

(a)

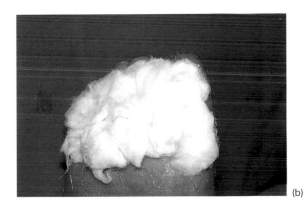

(b)

Fig. 16.4 Formaldehyde soaks for the treatment of mosaic warts. Mosaic warts are notoriously difficult to treat and only 50% will respond. Twelve per cent formaldehyde solution soaks are sometimes effective. The normal skin must be protected with Vaseline (a) and the formaldehyde can be applied using cotton-wool soaks (b) or, on the heel, by dipping the affected area in a saucer of the solution. Five months later the warts had virtually disappeared.

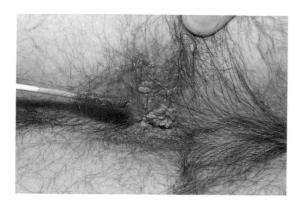

Fig. 16.5 Podophyllin treatment. Solutions range from 15 to 25% podophyllin. The warts are treated approximately once every 3 weeks. The solution should be washed off after 6–8 hours. If there is no response after six treatments, it is unlikely to be effective.

repeated treatments are commonly required. Mollusca contagiosa respond best to liquid nitrogen cryotherapy and a 10-second freeze is usually adequate (see Fig. 16.1). Common hand warts are treated with freeze times ranging from 10 to 30 seconds (Fig. 17.2). Current advice suggests that optimum treatment is achieved by cryotherapy once every 3 weeks, which results in a 75% cure rate after 12 weeks (four treatments). Combining salicylic acid/lactic acid treatment and liquid nitrogen therapy increases cure rates from 70 to 80%.

Between 40 and 80% of plantar warts respond to cryotherapy and the cure rate is increased by doing two rather than a single freeze–thaw cycle. Cryotherapy on the feet can, however, produce disabling painful blisters (Fig. 16.6) and may also produce permanent painful scars on the weight-bearing parts of the foot. Patients need to be aware of these shortcomings before starting treatment. Plane warts are difficult to treat with any modality, including cryotherapy; multiple applications are frequently necessary.

Table 16.4 Treatment options.

	First option	Second option	Third option	Fourth option
Common finger warts	Leave untreated Two thirds go within 2 years	Keratolytic	Cryotherapy	Curettage of periungual warts
Solitary face warts	Leave untreated Two thirds go in 2 years	Curettage	Cryotherapy	
Plane warts	Leave untreated	0.5% salicylic acid in olive oil	Topical retinoic acid	Cryotherapy
Genital warts	Always treat. Refer to genitourinary medicine clinic Podophyllin	Cryotherapy	Curettage	Laser destruction
Mosaic warts	Attempt to treat because of cross-infection risk Salicylic acid	Formaldehyde soaks	Cryotherapy	Podophyllin
Plantar warts	Leave untreated	Salicylic acid	Cryotherapy	Curettage of solitary warts
Molluscum contagiosum	Leave untreated 90% last < 1 year	Cryotherapy	Phenol pricking	

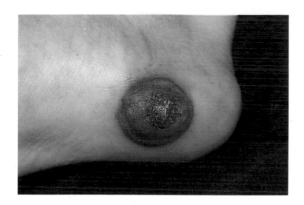

Fig. 16.6 Cryotherapy blister. Overtreatment with cryotherapy has caused a large haemorrhagic blister to appear on this patient's foot. Cryotherapy causes a lot of morbidity and a painful foot is very disabling. Warn the patient of these hazards before starting.

Curettage

Curettage of warts, like all therapies, is not totally effective. The treatment is painful and there is a risk of scarring and recurrence. Curettage should only be used when other methods have been unsuccessful. Solitary warts on the face of adults can usually be removed rapidly and effectively using curettage (Fig. 9.2). Plantar warts may be removed by curettage but the local anaesthetic injections are painful and recurrences can be a problem since patients are unlikely to want repeat treatment. Curettage is probably justifiable in painful solitary warts that have not responded to other therapies. On the sole there is always the risk of permanent, potentially painful scar formation and the patient should be warned of this possibility. There is a high risk of recurrence if mosaic warts are treated by curettage and this has considerable morbidity. Periungual warts are particularly difficult warts to curette off successfully but curettage may be a last resort. The nail frequently has to be removed to allow full curettage to be done. Multiple finger warts should not be treated by curettage unless all else has failed. Genital or perianal warts that have not responded to cryotherapy or podophyllin can be curetted off. It may be difficult to get a plane of cleavage in the soft friable skin and fulguration or incising the wart margin (Fig. 9.3) before curettage may be necessary.

Other therapies

Intralesional bleomycin, topical 5% 5-fluorouracil in dimethylsulphoxide, interferon and contact sensitizers have all been tried. Bleomycin injections are extremely painful; local anaesthetic is required and there is a risk of digital vasospasm, which may persist after treatment. Carbon dioxide laser therapy has been used. The treatment appears to be little more than an expensive form of cautery but may be more tissue-sparing since the extent of wart virus infection is believed to be more easily identified by the tissue response to laser therapy.

Immune-compromised patients

Patients on long-term immune suppression, particularly organ transplant recipients and human immunodeficiency virus (HIV)-infected individuals, are particularly vulnerable to widespread wart infections. All treatments can be tried but none is entirely successful because of the rate of reinfection. Oral retinoids may be tried if not otherwise contraindicated. Treatment is best limited to controlling rather than clearing the infection.

Practice points

• Cure should be judged by an expert using a magnifying glass and examination light to confirm reappearance of normal skin-ridge markings. Recurrence rates are higher when cure is decided by the patient, presumably because the warts never went in the first place.
• For salicylic acid treatment to be successful it is essential that the patient understands how to use the treatment properly and is expertly supervised (Table 16.2).
• There are always a proportion of treatment failures. Approximately 30% of hand, 20% of simple plantar and 50% of mosaic wart patients fail to respond.

- Children with foot warts should wear a protective rubber sock when they go swimming to prevent cross-infection.
- Because of the high spontaneous remission rates, painful therapies are rarely justified in children.

Further reading

Berth-Jones J, Bourke J, Eglitis H *et al.* (1994) Value of a second freeze–thaw cycle in cryotherapy of common warts. *Br J Dermatol* **131**: 883–886.

Bunney MH, Benton C & Cubie H (1992) *Viral Warts, Biology and Treatment*. Oxford University Press, Oxford.

Bunney MH, Nolan MW & Williams DA (1976) An assessment of methods of treating viral warts by comparative treatment trials based on a standard design. *Br J Dermatol* **94**: 667–679.

Highet AS & Kurtz J (1992) Viral infections. In: Champion RH, Burton JL & Ebling FJG (eds) *Textbook of Dermatology*, 5th edition. Blackwell Science, Oxford.

Williams HC, Pottier A & Strachan D (1993) The descriptive epidemiology of warts in British school children. *Br J Dermatol* **128**: 504–511.

17: Cryotherapy in general practice

Freezing agents

Several methods of freezing skin are available (Table 17.1). These vary in their convenience, expense and the temperature achieved. It is suggested that cryotherapy produces cell damage by four mechanisms: (i) intracellular ice formation; (ii) osmotic effects, (iii) blood supply changes; and (iv) immune stimulation. Intracellular ice formation damages the cell. As the cell thaws the osmotic differences resulting from differential ice formation and hence reduced volume of water available for dissolved solutes disrupt cells. Small blood vessels are damaged by freezing, resulting in ischaemic damage, and finally disrupted cells release antigenic components which stimulate an immune response. The extent of injury is determined by the rate of freezing, the coldest temperature reached, the freeze time and the rate of thawing. Maximum damage is produced by rapid freezing and slow thawing. Repeating the freeze–thaw cycle produces much greater tissue damage than a single freeze because the greater conductivity of the previously frozen skin and the already impaired circulation both allow a greater and faster depth of cold penetration.

The temperature required to produce cell death is not established, although it is commonly recommended that a temperature of $-30°C$ at the deep and lateral borders is required. In practice it is not necessary to measure tissue temperatures achieved during cryotherapy as clinical studies have determined appropriate liquid nitrogen spray freeze times for common skin conditions (Table 17.2). Freeze times for other methods are longer because of the higher temperature. For example, freeze times for carbon dioxide snow

Table 17.1 Characteristics of available cryotherapy agents.

Method	Temperature achieved	Comments
Salt and ice	$-20°C$	Readily available, difficult to use, inadequate temperature
Dimethyl ether and propane (Histofreezer)	$-50°C$	Readily available, convenient, expensive
Nitrous oxide	$-70°C$	Fiddly, slow, expensive, cumbersome equipment
Carbon dioxide snow	$-79°C$	Fiddly, slow, easily portable, readily available
Liquid nitrogen	$-196°C$	Fast, convenient; reliable supply of liquid nitrogen has to be arranged

Table 17.2 Treatment times for skin lesions using liquid nitrogen.

Lesion	Freeze time	Margin of normal skin also frozen (mm)
Viral warts	Single freeze 10–30 seconds	1–2
Seborrhoeic warts	Single freeze 10–30 seconds	1–2
Actinic keratosis	Single freeze 5–20 seconds	1–2
Venous lake	Single freeze 10–30 seconds with pressure	1
Bowen's disease	Single 30-second freeze	2
Basal cell carcinoma	Two 30-second freezes, with 2-minute thaw time	3

Note: The duration of freeze varies depending on lesion thickness and response to previous cryotherapy.
These freeze times are based on the use of a Cryac spray with a C nozzle held 5 mm away from the skin.

treatment of warts are three times longer than those recommended with liquid nitrogen. There is little published work on the freeze times required for many of the agents listed and the remainder of this chapter will deal with liquid nitrogen cryotherapy as this is the best studied and most convenient method available, provided a supply of liquid nitrogen is readily available.

Indications

Liquid nitrogen cryotherapy is an effective, simple and inexpensive destructive therapy that can be used for the treatment of a wide range of benign and malignant lesions. There are two disadvantages of cryotherapy. First, as a destructive therapy no histological confirmation is obtained during treament; thus a missed diagnosis may go unnoticed. Second, it is painful and produces significant short-term morbidity. These disadvantages have to be weighed against its economy and speed. Manufacturers suggest that cryotherapy can be used to treat a range of lesions, including naevi, squamous cell carcinoma, dermatofibroma, cysts, etc. However, the results produced are variable and there is no confirmatory histological diagnosis. In dermatological practice these lesions are usually only frozen by those with a particular interest and expertise in cryotherapy and I would advise non-experts against the use of cryotherapy to treat such lesions.

Safety aspects

If liquid nitrogen is carried in a car it may leak out if the flask tips up. Sudden evaporation of liquid nitrogen creates a freezing nitrogen mist which could fill the car, obscure vision and, in theory, by displacing the air asphyxiate the driver. Thus, when liquid nitrogen is carried in a car, drive with the window open, transport only small volumes ($\leqslant 1$ litre), use a vacuum flask designed to carry liquid nitrogen and keep this upright in a specially designed carrying box. Since liquid nitrogen evaporates away continuously there always has to be a vent hole in the flask to allow the nitrogen gas to escape; without a vent the gas pressure would cause an explosion. When pouring liquid nitrogen, protective gloves and face mask should be worn to guard against splashes. If liquid nitrogen is stored it must be kept in an adequately ventilated area — usually a secure outside cage. Evaporation can be reduced by storage in a pressurized container, although these are expensive.

Equipment

• **Essential:** liquid nitrogen, suitable vacuum flask and transporting box.
• **Optional:** Dewar flask to store liquid nitrogen, liquid nitrogen spray.

Liquid nitrogen is inexpensive but since the liquid is at $-196\,^{\circ}$C it constantly evaporates away even when stored in a cold room. Twenty five litres of liquid nitrogen held in a vented non-pressurized Dewar flask will evaporate away in approximately 10 days. For large general practices direct supply may be an option. If liquid nitrogen is stored a secure, ventilated site and storage flask will be required. It is more practical to arrange for a small regular supply of liquid nitrogen (2 litres is ample) and bring patients to a cryotherapy clinic once a month or so. Liquid nitrogen may be obtained from a hospital pharmacy, pathology or university laboratories and industrial users. Control of substances harmful or hazardous (COSHH) regulations do not preclude the carriage of small quantities of liquid nitrogen in a private vehicle.

Freeze time

The freeze times discussed in this book begin at the moment the target area of skin is completely frozen i.e. when the whole target area looks white (the ice ball). Thereafter liquid nitrogen is trickled on to the target area to maintain the ice ball at the required margin. Liquid nitrogen spray is halted when the freeze time is up. Thus, for example to produce a 20-second freeze time, the target area will first have to be frozen by spraying with liquid nitrogen for 5–10 seconds or more. Once the whole target area is frozen white, the freeze time measurement is started. Liquid nitrogen spray is then sprayed intermittently or trickled on to the target area for 20 seconds to maintain the ice ball. When 20 seconds is up the spraying stops but it takes the skin another 15 seconds or so to thaw out.

Cryotherapy of viral warts

A liquid nitrogen spray (Fig. 17.1) is easy to operate, convenient and fast, but relatively expensive. A simple alternative is to hold and transport the liquid nitrogen in a suitably vented and boxed vacuum flask and apply it using a cotton-wool bud applicator.

Indications

Viruses are not killed by cold temperatures; cryotherapy works by destroying the infected tissue. In the majority of patients warts heal spontaneously, painlessly and without scarring in time. Other remedies should be considered (Chapter 16). Liquid nitrogen cryotherapy is very painful and thus inappropriate for the treatment of children's warts. Liquid nitrogen cryotherapy cures approximately 75% of patients after 4 treatments given at 3-weekly intervals.

Technique

Cotton bud method. The aim is to produce a blister a little bigger than the wart, this causes the wart to separate from the underlying dermis (Fig. 17.2). The bud should be large enough to hold a small quantity of liquid nitrogen within the cotton fibres. The size of the skin-contact area can be adjusted by manipulating the end of the bud before it is dipped into the liquid nitrogen. The end of the cotton bud can then be precisely applied to the wart; skill and practice are required to do this properly. No pressure is required and should be avoided, as this will produce a deeper freeze and more extensive local damage. A rim of normal tissue (Fig. 17.2) should also be frozen

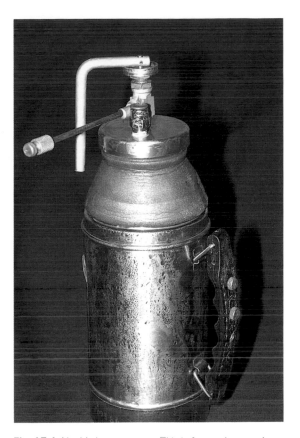

Fig. 17.1 Liquid nitrogen spray. This is fast and convenient. If you use a lot of liquid nitrogen therapy it might be a worthwhile investment. Small quantities of liquid nitrogen can be transported in this type of flask, provided it is kept upright. A full unused 3-litre canister, kept at room temperature, will evaporate completely away in 10–12 hours. Thus, in practice the flask has to be filled on the day it is going to be used.

around the wart (Table 17.3). The required freeze time is measured from the moment the ice ball covers the wart and rim of surrounding normal skin, thus 15–20 seconds of liquid nitrogen application might be required to produce a 10-second freeze time. It is important not to contaminate the liquid nitrogen with skin fragments containing wart virus by using the same applicator for different individuals.

Freeze times of up to 20 seconds can readily be achieved using the cotton bud technique. To avoid contaminating the liquid nitrogen a small

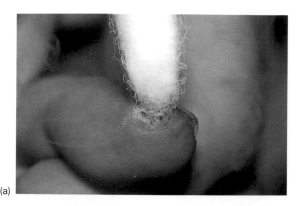

(a)

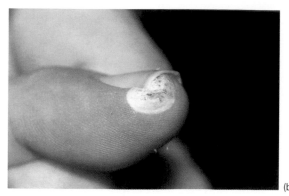

(b)

Fig. 17.2 Liquid nitrogen application using a cotton-wool bud. Viral warts that have failed to respond to medical therapies can be treated using liquid nitrogen cryotherapy. The cotton bud is dipped into the liquid nitrogen and the drop of liquid nitrogen on the end applied to the wart (a). Do not press down firmly with the cotton bud as this may produce an unnecessarily deep freeze. Flick off excessive amounts of liquid on the bud before starting, to avoid it dripping on to the patient. Ensure that a rim of normal skin is also frozen around the wart (b). Approximately 75% of patients with viral warts are cured after a total of 4 treatments given once every 3 weeks. Do not dip the applicator back into liquid nitrogen because hepatitis B, herpes simplex and wart viruses all survive liquid nitrogen immersion. Pour a small quantity into a disposable polystyrene beaker if the applicator needs to be recharged during treatment.

quantity can be poured into a disposable polystyrene cup and this can be used to recharge the cotton bud for the same patient.

Liquid nitrogen spray method. A liquid nitrogen spray (Fig. 16.1, Fig. 17.1) is faster, more precise and colder temperatures can be achieved for longer. This last advantage is important in the treatment of skin cancer but not relevant when treating benign lesions. When recording the cryosurgery procedure, note the duration of freeze, size and distance from the skin of the nozzle used, as this information will help to demonstrate sound technique if problems occur (Table 17.3).

Table 17.3 Freezing technique.

Decide how long a freeze time is required
Identify target area to be frozen to include the lesion plus a margin of normal skin (Table 17.2)
Begin spraying with liquid nitrogen. Start timing when the target area is completely frozen
Continue spraying with liquid nitrogen in shorter bursts to maintain ice-ball formation within the target area
Stop spraying when the freeze time is up
Record freeze time, nozzle size and distance from the skin

Cryotherapy of seborrhoeic warts

Symptomatic or disfiguring seborrhoeic warts can be readily destroyed using liquid nitrogen. Freeze times of 10–20 seconds are usually effective and this can be repeated 3–4 weeks later if necessary.

Cryotherapy of vascular lesions

Vascular abnormalities such as venous lakes or Campbell de Morgan spots can be treated with cryotherapy. The blood should be squeezed out before cryotherapy is attempted. This can be done using special cryoprobes of various sizes. A simple and inexpensive alternative is to compress out the blood using a spoon curette and freeze the skin by squirting liquid nitrogen on to the curette whilst this is pressed on to the skin (Fig. 17.3).

Cryotherapy of actinic keratoses

Solitary or larger hypertrophic actinic keratoses can be treated with a variety of therapies, including liquid nitrogen (Fig. 17.4). Careful diagnosis is essential to exclude basal or squamous cell carci-

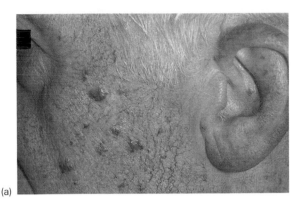

(a)

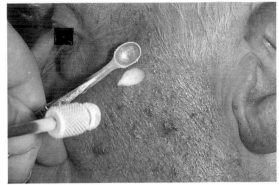

(b)

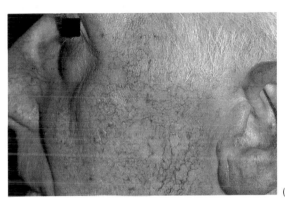

(c)

Fig. 17.3 Cryotherapy of venous lakes. Benign vascular lesions such as venous lakes (a) respond well to cryotherapy. Vascular lesions are best frozen when blood flow through the area is excluded, thereby removing the warming effect of local blood flow. Local pressure is the simplest method for reducing flow. Alternatively, simply freezing the end of a suitable-sized spoon curette (b) by spraying with liquid nitrogen before and during skin application is equally effective, faster and more varied-shaped lesions can be treated. The result 2 months later (c), after two treatments, shows that most of the venous lakes had been destroyed.

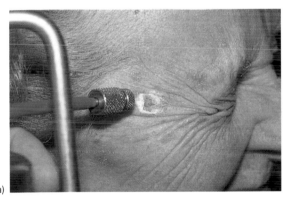

(a)

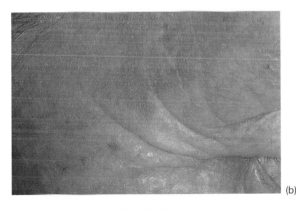

(b)

Fig. 17.4 Cryotherapy of actinic keratoses. Solitary actinic keratoses can be effectively treated with liquid nitrogen therapy delivered from a liquid nitrogen spray (a) or cotton bud, as only a short freeze time is required. A single 15–30-second freeze will produce sufficient epidermal damage to destroy the dysplastic epidermis. Large keratoses may require several treatments given at 4–6-week intervals. Two months after one treatment the keratosis was destroyed and the scar barely visible (b).

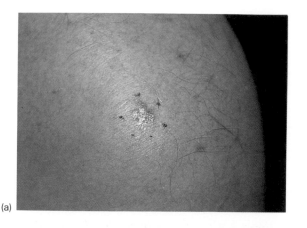
(a)

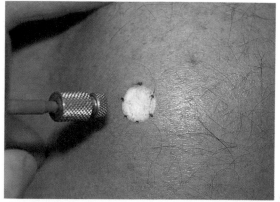
(b)

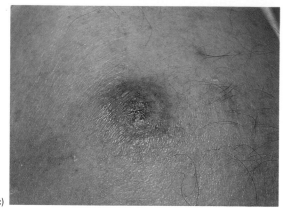
(c)

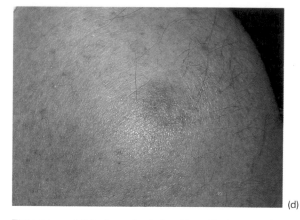
(d)

Fig. 17.5 Cryotherapy of basal cell carcinoma on the shoulder. A 3-mm margin of normal skin is marked around the tumour (a). The entire area was frozen and the ice ball maintained within the marked area for 30 seconds by trickling the liquid nitrogen over the target area (b).

The area was left to thaw slowly for at least 2 minutes and the freeze was then reapplied to achieve a further 30-second freeze. One week later the treated site was red and swollen (c). Appearance at 2 months (d).

noma prior to treatment as the freeze times used will not eradicate these tumours. Widespread actinic keratoses are best treated using other therapies, including 5-fluorouracil therapy (Fig. 18.7).

Cryotherapy of basal cell carcinoma

Liquid nitrogen can be used to destroy basal cell carcinomas, although this should only be performed by an adequately trained and experienced individual and is not a generally recommended procedure for general practice. Therapy is much more aggressive than that used for benign lesions (Fig. 17.5). Accurate diagnosis before treatment

is essential because histological material is not obtained. The best results are achieved by selecting only small (< 10 mm diameter), well-defined tumours at non-critical sites. Attempts to treat large, ill-defined, invasive, morphoeic or recurrent tumours result in poorer cure rates. Tumours at sites associated with a high recurrence rate, including the side of the nose, behind and in front of the ear, should be avoided. A 3-mm margin of normal skin should also be included in the area treated. The tumour must be treated for two 30-second freeze times with a 2-minute thaw time in between. Treatment is thus painful and profound skin and tumour necrosis occurs.

During cryotherapy, freeze spreads laterally more readily than deeply. It cannot be assumed that a hemisphere of tissue has been frozen the radius of the ice ball. If a deeply seated tumour is treated, longer freeze times and margins of uninvolved skin must be used. Such treatments should only be attempted by an experienced operator.

Practice points

• Normal immediate reactions after liquid nitrogen cryotherapy include pain (Fig. 17.4), inflammation, redness, swelling and blistering. Warn your patient of the consequences and use the word 'burn' when describing the reaction, so that patients will know what to expect. A brief written note outlining the consequences of treatment may be useful (Table 17.4).

• Inflammation after cryotherapy is thought to be prostaglandin-mediated and can be reduced by applying clobetasol propionate cream (twice daily for 4 days) or aspirin (300 mg/day) therapy.

• Keratin and crust may insulate the tumour and prevent adequate freezing. When possible, remove these before cryosurgery. In the treatment of warts, the keratin thickness should be reduced by the patient treating the wart in between cryotherapy treatments by using a keratolytic and paring (see page 102).

• Serious late complications of freezing warts on the backs of the fingers include extensor tendon rupture. This is exceedingly rare but may occur if a long freeze is used and the freeze penetrates deeply. When freezing a wart on the dorsum of the fingers, manipulate the skin to ensure that the frozen skin does not become attached to the underlying tendon. The depth of freeze can also be finely tuned by directing the spray obliquely rather than vertically down on to the wart.

• Nerve damage resulting in motor or sensory loss may also occur. Vulnerable sites include the lateral aspect of the knee over the head of the fibula (common peroneal nerve), elbow (ulnar nerve) and fingers where freezing over the lateral palmar aspect may damage the palmar digital nerve and produce distal sensory loss.

• Scarring can occur with liquid nitrogen if the freeze time is prolonged. This is particularly important around the matrix area of the nail where nail distortion may occur, and in hair-bearing areas where a permanent bald patch may result. Such scarring is not uncommon after tumour treatment when prolonged and aggressive cryosurgery is used but will not occur with freeze times of 10 seconds or less. Freezing non-responding warts for longer than 30 seconds produces little further therapeutic effect and increases the risk of damage to normal tissues.

• Cells are more susceptible to cold injury than supporting structures. Melanocytes are particularly sensitive and depigmentation — often

Table 17.4 Patient information sheet after cryotherapy (freezing) of warts.

Your wart has been frozen. The treated area will be painful for several hours and it will swell. If blisters form, these may be burst with a sterile needle but do not apply any ointments or creams unless prescribed by your doctor. Pain and swelling may be reduced by aspirin therapy if you are able to take this drug. Cryotherapy frequently needs to be repeated so do not be surprised if further treatments are required

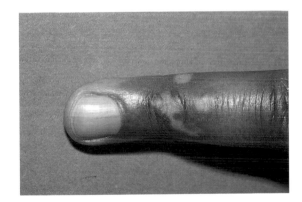

Fig. 17.6 Pigment changes in black skin after cryotherapy. This hypopigmentation occurred after one cryotherapy treatment for viral warts. Melanocytes are particularly vulnerable to cold damage. Hypo- or hyperpigmentation is common after liquid nitrogen therapy. After a short single freeze, repigmentation usually occurs but hypopigmentation may be permanent after cryotherapy for skin cancer.

permanent — can be expected following treatment of malignancies. Patients with black or brown skin commonly develop hypo- or hyperpigmentation at skin injury sites, particularly after cryotherapy. Warn such patients of these risks and only use cryotherapy on the face of black people as a last resort (Fig. 17.6).

• Cryotherapy on a lower limb is likely to result in ulceration, particularly if there is associated peripheral vascular disease. This is particularly important when considering using cryotherapy for the treatment of Bowen's disease on the leg.

• Large areas, i.e. greater than 2 cm diameter, can usually only be frozen for longer than 20 seconds if the area is treated as several 1.5–2 cm diameter adjacent and overlapping sites. These areas can be marked with pen before starting treatment to ensure the whole area is treated.

Further reading

Colver G, Jackson A & Dawber RPR (1992) *Cutaneous Cryosurgery*. Martin Dunitz, London.

Faber WR, Naafs B & Sillevis Smitt JH (1987) Sensory loss following cryosurgery of skin lesions. *Br J Dermatol* **117**: 343–347.

Holt PJA (1988) Cryotherapy for skin cancer: results over a 5 year period using liquid nitrogen spray cryosurgery. *Br J Dermatol* **119**: 231–240.

Kuflik EG (1994) Cryosurgery updated. *J Am Acad Dermatol* **31**: 925–944.

Kuflik EG & Gage AA (1991) The 5 year cure rate achieved by cryosurgery for skin cancer. *J Am Acad Dermatol* **24**: 1002–1004.

Neel HB, Ketcham AS & Hammond WG (1971) Requisites for successful cryogenic surgery of cancer. *Arch Surg* **102**: 45–48.

Torre D (1986) Cryosurgery of basal cell carcinoma. *J Am Acad Dermatol* **15**: 917–929.

18: Treatment of skin tumours

This chapter discusses the management of common skin tumours (basal cell carcinoma (BCC), squamous cell carcinoma (SCC), keratoacanthoma) and premalignant dermatoses (Bowen's disease and actinic keratoses) seen in general and dermatological practice.

Basal cell carcinoma

Principle of treatment — select the appropriate technique for the tumour type

All treatments of BCC can be expected to result in cure rates in excess of 95%, provided the appropriate technique has been selected for the tumour and the treatment is performed by a skilled and experienced operator. Recurrences occur more frequently if poor technique is employed or the wrong types of treatment are selected for the type of BCC being treated. The various techniques have different attributes and not all are appropriate for every tumour (Table 18.1). For example, curettage has little place in the treatment of an infiltrating BCC recurring after excision. Curettage is generally reserved for small well-defined BCCs on sites that can be readily treated (see Table 9.2).

Excision margins

When treating patients with skin cancer, it is imperative not to compromise the adequacy of the excision to make the repair easier. A margin of apparently uninvolved skin must be removed with the tumour to guard against the possibility of the tumour extending beyond the visible margin. Subclinical extension and risk of recurrence vary with the size, histological type, site and previous treatment of BCC being treated. Thus, high-risk tumours require wider excision margins

(Table 18.2). The margins suggested are however only a guide and, with the exception of well-defined BCCs, have not been arrived at by rigorous scentific study. Wide margins may mean unnecessary removal of uninvolved skin and do not preclude the possibility that a small tongue of tumour extends beyond the margin. In most situations where wide margins are recommended, microscopically controlled excision of the tumour (Mohs surgery; see below) provides a more rational and potentially tissue-sparing approach than blind wide margin excision.

Recurrent tumours and Mohs surgery

BCCs which recur do so at different intervals depending on the method of treatment (Fig. 18.1). Recurrent tumours are more difficult to cure following retreatment than primary tumours (Fig. 18.2). For example, if a recurrence following radiotherapy is treated with more radiotherapy, approximately 25% recur. The recurrence rate after attempted single complete excision of recurrent BCCs is on average 13%. Similarly, curettage of recurrences produces a 60% recurrence rate. Some recurrent tumours are initially undertreated because they spread beyond the visible margin. The situation is further complicated by the initial incomplete excision and repair, which may result in residual tumour being left at separate sites in the skin. In these circumstances any technique that depends on a visual assessment of the tumour extent is unlikely to work. To overcome this difficulty Fred Mohs, an American surgeon, developed a technique that attempts to follow the tumour extent histologically with the aim of completely excising residual tumour fragments invisible to the naked eye after the visible bulk of tumour has been removed (Fig. 18.3). The technique has become widely accepted as the

Table 18.1 Attributes of different techniques for the treatment of basal cell carcinoma (BCC).

Technique	Attributes	Weaknesses	Indications	Contraindications
Curettage and cautery	Simple technique Quick Effective when used appropriately	Deceptively simple Easily done incorrectly or used inappropriately Scarring unpredictable	Small well-defined BCC on appropriate sites	Recurrences Large tumours (> 20 mm) Ill-defined tumours Morphoeic BCCs Incorrect sites (Table 9.3)
Cryotherapy	Simple Inexpensive Effective	Deceptively simple Easily done incorrectly or used inappropriately Painful Great morbidity No histology	Small well-defined BCCs on appropriate sites	Large tumours (> 20 mm diameter) Ill-defined BCCs Morphoeic tumours Recurrent tumours
Attempted complete excision	Histological confirmation Cosmesis potentially excellent Rapid healing	Time-consuming	All types of tumour	When surgery is deforming and alternatives produce potentially better cosmetic results, e.g. ear Tumours with ill-defined edges Recurrent BCCs
Radiotherapy	No surgery Good cosmesis with multiple fractionated doses	Scars get worse with time Poor cosmesis after single fractionated dose Risk of radiation necrosis Risk of radiotherapy-induced tumours Recurrences appear up to 10–15 years later Prolonged follow-up required	Surgery not acceptable Sites where surgery potentially deforming, e.g. lip and eyelid	Ill-defined BCCs Morphoeic tumours Recurrent tumours Basal cell naevus syndrome patients Young patients (risk of radiotherapy-induced skin tumours and skin necrosis) Xeroderma pigmentosa patients Sites where radiotherapy damage is unacceptable, e.g. over lacrimal gland
Mohs surgery (microscopically controlled excision)	Histological confirmation of tumour excision High cure rates Tissue-sparing	Time-consuming More than one operation required	Recurrent tumours Ill-defined tumours Sites with high recurrence rates	Unnecessary in small primary or well-defined BCCs
Topical 5-fluorouracil	No surgery Easy for the doctor Inexpensive Good cosmesis Useful on keloid-prone sites	Limited usefulness Slow Messy Causes morbidity	Only used on superficial BCCs on the trunk	All other BCCs

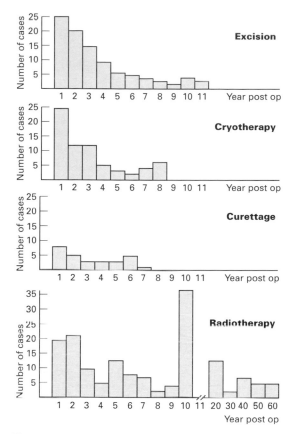

Fig. 18.1 Consequences of incomplete basal cell carcinoma (BCC) excision. Recurrences appear after different intervals depending on the initial treatment. Adapted from Emmett AJ (1990) Surgical analysis and biological behaviour of 2277 basal cell carcinomas. *Aust NZ J Surg* **60**: 855–863, with permission.

treatment of choice for difficult tumours following reported 5-year cure rates of 98% for primary tumours and 96% for recurrences.

Second-intention healing

Wounds created by curettage or shave excision of benign lesions are left to heal spontaneously and frequently produce excellent cosmetic results. Wounds created after tumour excision can also be left to heal by second intention. The technique is simple (Fig. 18.4) and effective when used appropriately. Care must be taken to choose wounds where the cosmetic result will be satisfactory.

Table 18.2 Excision margins recommended for different types of basal cell carcinoma (BCC).

Type of BCC	Recommended excision margin (mm)
Clinical type	
Well-defined nodular BCCs	3–4
Recurrent tumours	10
Ill-defined tumour	6
Histological types	
Common solid	3–4
Morphoeic pattern	6–8
Infiltrative multifocal type	8–10
Metatypical	8–10

Good results are achieved on the nasolabial fold, medial canthus, scalp and pre- and postauricular skin (Fig. 18.5). Approximately 45% of the healing that occurs does so by contraction of the wound and stretching of the surrounding tissues. Thus, defects adjacent to mobile skin edges such as the lip or nasal rim may result in distortion of these free margins and wounds at these sites are rarely left to heal by second intention (Table 18.3).

Table 18.3 Secondary-intention healing

	Good response	Poor response
Site	Medial canthus	Nose tip
	Temple	Around the lip
	Nasolabial fold	Partial-thickness
	Scalp	lower eyelid
	Preauricular area	Exposed bone
	Postauricular area	
	Full-thickness lower	
	eyelid	
	Exposed perichondrium	
Patient type	Older patients	Young patients
	Cooperative and	Black skin — risk of
	motivated	keloids may be
		greater
Size	Any size	
Tumour type	Any	

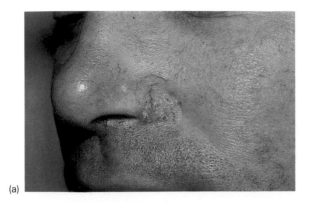

(a)

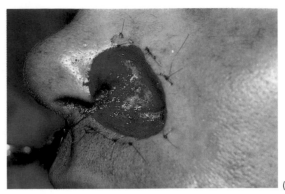

(b)

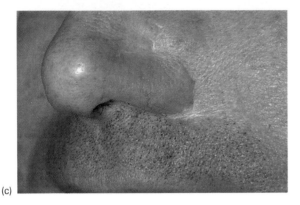

(c)

Fig. 18.2 Recurrent basal cell carcinoma (BCC). This recurrent BCC (a) was completely excised using horizontal margins for tumour margin control, resulting in removal of most of the ala of the nose (b). Subsequent expert plastic surgical repair produced an excellent cosmetic result (c).

Technique

The tumour is excised with an appropriate margin of normal skin. The specimen can be oriented with a marking suture at one pole and a note made of the specimen orientation. Haemostasis is achieved with electrodesiccation (Chaper 5). The wound dressing should be covered by a pressure dressing at least for the first 24 hours. The dressing should be changed at 2–4-day intervals, depending on the wound size and amount of exudate. Wounds can be cleaned with a simple antiseptic such as 10 vol hydrogen peroxide, an antiseptic ointment applied (e.g. Polyfax, Flamazine or Betadine ointment) and the wound covered with a simple non-adherent dressing held in place with adhesive tape. By 7 days the histology result should be available and the adequacy or otherwise of the excision confirmed. If the tumour has been incompletely excised the margin can be re-excised 1–2 weeks after the first exci-

sion. The technique does not provide the same complete excision margin control as the horizontal sections of Mohs surgery (Fig. 18.3) since vertical sections are taken and the entire excision margin is not examined.

Once full excision has been confirmed, the wound can be allowed to heal. The dressing will need to be changed three to four times a week or more frequently initially and this can be done by the patient or nurse. On each occasion the wound is cleaned with hydrogen peroxide to remove any crust or debris, a thin smear of antiseptic ointment applied and the wound covered by a small dressing. On average a 25 mm diameter head and neck wound takes approximately 35 days to heal.

Complications

These wounds are surprisingly painfree (Table 18.4). Infections are uncommon but when present are characterized by redness and swelling

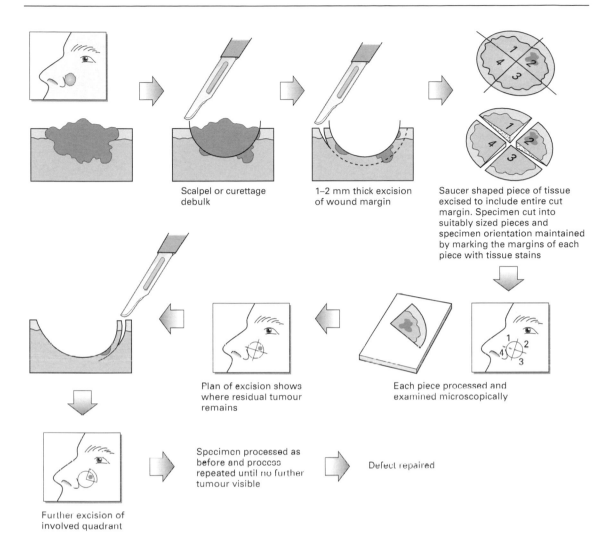

Scalpel or curettage debulk

1–2 mm thick excision of wound margin

Saucer shaped piece of tissue excised to include entire cut margin. Specimen cut into suitably sized pieces and specimen orientation maintained by marking the margins of each piece with tissue stains

Plan of excision shows where residual tumour remains

Each piece processed and examined microscopically

Further excision of involved quadrant

Specimen processed as before and process repeated until no further tumour visible

Defect repaired

Fig. 18.3 Management of difficult skin tumours using micrographic surgery (Mohs surgery). The clinically evident tumour is excised or curetted off. A margin of apparently normal skin 1–2 mm thick is then excised around the complete margin of the wound, including the deep surface. This is cut up into smaller pieces, usually less than 1 cm diameter, and these are each processed and examined separately and horizontal sections taken so that the entire excision margin is examined. The wound and specimen have to be carefully marked so that the site of each piece can be identified. If tumour is present in one or some of the specimens, further excisions are performed until there is no visible tumour at the excision margins. The wound then has to be closed by whatever method is considered likely to give the best result. If skin sections are examined using frozen sections, the whole process can be completed in a day. If formalin-fixed and paraffin-embedded skin sections are used, the patient has to return at 24–48-hour intervals for each stage of the procedure. Paraffin sections produce much better histological sections. The technique is only appropriate for tumours that spread by continuous extension. It is thus not suitable for melanoma.

of the surrounding skin. A yellow exudate is common in the first few weeks and on its own is not a sign of infection. Exposed bone and cartilage must be carefully dressed to ensure that they do not desiccate and ultimately necrose. This risk disappears once the area is covered by granulation tissue. Over-granulation will respond to topical steroid application.

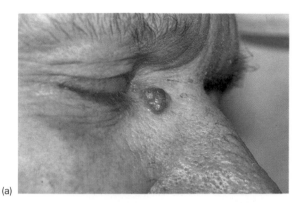

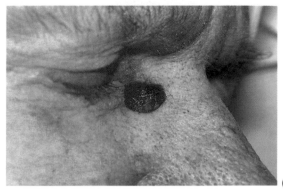

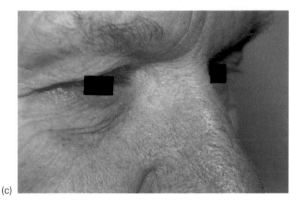

Fig. 18.4 Second-intention healing. This medial canthus basal cell carcinoma (a) was excised (b) and the wound allowed to heal by second intention. The cosmetic result 2 years later was excellent (c).

Incompletely excised tumours

Approximately a third of incompletely excised BCCs recur. Thus, a histologically incompletely excised BCC should be re-excised if it could spread to involve an adjacent cosmetically or functionally important structure, e.g. the eyelid. As the BCC was probably originally incompletely excised because the tumour extended beyond the visible margin, it is essential to check the tumour margin extent histologically to avoid a large area of normal skin being unnecessarily excised or tumour being accidentally left behind. The Mohs surgical excision technique is thus an ideal method to be used in this situation (Fig. 18.3). Postoperative radiotherapy can also be tried although, since it is impossible to know how wide a field to treat, results are less good. Incompletely excised BCCs at other sites, e.g. the back, can reasonably be left untreated and followed up yearly since if they recur, wider excision is un-

likely to cause difficulty. When faced with this type of dilemma it is best to discuss the problem with the patient and allow him/her to make an informed choice.

Malignant melanoma

Patients with a pigmented lesion characteristic of a melanoma should be sent for an urgent specialist opinion. More commonly, however, the mole appears benign, but complete reassurance cannot be given. Before surgery, carefully examine the

Table 18.4 Advantages and disadvantages of secondary-intention healing.

Advantages	Disadvantages
Simple	Slow healing phase
Recurrences easily identified	Dressing required
Painless	Scar unpredictable
Quick initial surgery	

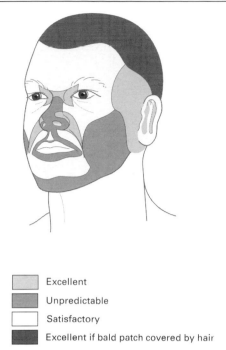

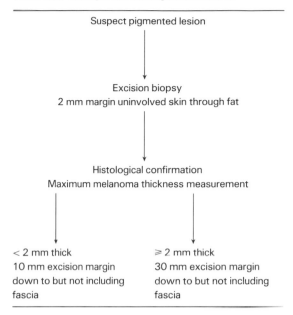

Table 18.5 Management of malignant melanoma.

Suspect pigmented lesion
↓
Excision biopsy
2 mm margin uninvolved skin through fat
↓
Histological confirmation
Maximum melanoma thickness measurement

< 2 mm thick	≥ 2 mm thick
10 mm excision margin down to but not including fascia	30 mm excision margin down to but not including fascia

■ Excellent

■ Unpredictable

□ Satisfactory

■ Excellent if bald patch covered by hair

Fig. 18.5 Effect of site on cosmetic result of second intention healing. In general, the medial canthus, nasolabial fold, temple, periauricular skin and concave areas of the ear do predictably well. Wounds on the lower eyelid can be left to heal spontaneously, provided they are full-thickness, i.e. the tarsal plate and conjunctiva are also excised with the skin. If only skin is excised, there is a risk of ectropion. On the scalp the scars are approximately half the size of the wound and provided they are covered by the hair are invisible. Adapted from Zitelli JA (1983) Wound healing by secondary intention. *J Am Acad Dermatol* **9**: 407–415, with permission.

suspect lesion so that it will be possible to correlate the clinical and histological features. First, note whether the mole is palpable; tumours thicker than 2 mm invariably are. Second, look for tumour ulceration as this is associated with a worse prognosis. Examine the patient for local, in-transit and distant metastases.

Suspect naevi can be excised down to fat with a 2-mm margin of normal skin (Chapter 13) and the result and histology reviewed 7–10 days later. If the lesion proves to be a melanoma the patient can be referred urgently for further surgery. No harm will have been done since a similar biopsy would normally be undertaken prior to curative surgery (Table 18.5). Avoid incisional biopsy of suspicious pigmented lesions; this may be associated with early lymphatic spread; it interferes with histological measurement of maximal tumour thickness, the single most important prognostic indicator, and there is also a risk of sample error with localized malignant change going unrecognized. Definitive melanoma excision should ideally be done as soon as possible. There are no studies relating delay in excision with outcome. A current UK study of melanoma excision allows for the second definitive excision to be done within 45 days of the initial excision biopsy.

Excision margin size depends on melanoma thickness (Table 18.5). The precise best method of management is still evolving and further large prospective studies are required. The current advice is to remove a 10 mm margin of normal skin down to, but not including, fascia for thin (< 2 mm thick) melanomas and a 30 mm margin for thicker tumours. These guidelines will change as further evidence becomes available. For example, preliminary evidence suggests that 2 mm margins for thin (i.e. < 0.75 mm thick) melanomas are as good as 10 mm margins. Furthermore,

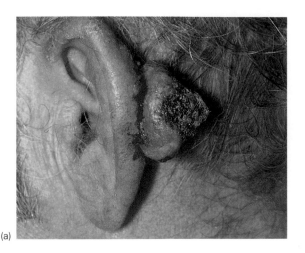

(a)

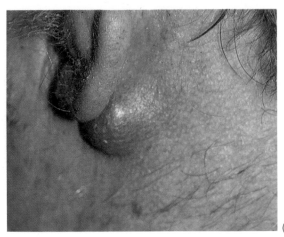

(b)

Fig. 18.6 Metastasis of a squamous cell carcinoma. This large squamous cell carcinoma on the ear (a) metastasized to a draining lymph node 2 months after excision (b).

there is controversy about the wisdom of narrow margins for tumours 1–2 mm thick and a study comparing the outcome of 10 mm versus 30 mm margin excisions for melanomas > 2 mm thick is in progress. Prospective removal of draining lymph nodes is sometimes also done in melanomas > 1.5 mm thick if a single lymphatic drainage pathway exists. This technique however is not widely practised as the morbidity is considerable and the effectiveness is not fully established.

Squamous cell carcinoma and keratoacanthoma

Most SCCs that arise on sun-damaged skin are relatively innocuous tumours with a low prevalence of metastasis. By contrast, SCCs that arise on non-sun-damaged skin, and lip and ear tumours, are more likely to metastasize early to draining lymph nodes (Fig. 18.6). The potentially fatal outcome of SCC means that these tumours should always be treated early and adequately. Prospective study of subclinical microscopic tumour extension suggests that 6 mm margins are required when excising large (> 20 mm diameter), histologically aggressive and high-risk site

tumours, whereas 4 mm margins are adequate for other SCC types.

Keratoacanthomas are classically symmetrical, rapidly growing, keratinizing tumours, with a shoulder of stretched, normal skin and a central keratin plug. These tumours reach their maximum size in 3 months and then begin to resolve spontaneously. Aggressive SCCs can appear almost identical and thus if there is any doubt about the diagnosis the tumour should be treated as a squamous cell carcinoma.

Bowen's disease and actinic keratoses

Approximately a third of patients with actinic keratoses show evidence of spontaneous resolution of at least one actinic keratosis after a year of sun avoidance. Thus, it is worthwhile advising patients with extensive sun damage to protect themselves from further sun exposure. Less than 1% of actinic keratoses develop into SCCs and the tumours that arise are believed to be relatively innocuous and rarely metastasize (< 5%). Multiple actinic keratoses are best treated by liquid nitrogen cryotherapy and solitary lesions can be curetted off. Topical 5-fluorouracil (5FU, Efudix) is an effective if somewhat irritant therapy. Experience in the method of application and likely outcome is essential. Lesions that fail to respond to 5FU or cryotherapy should be scrutinized for possible invasive SCC development (Fig. 18.7).

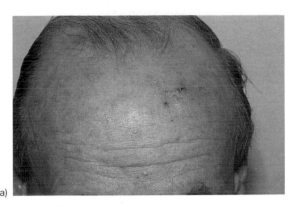
(a)

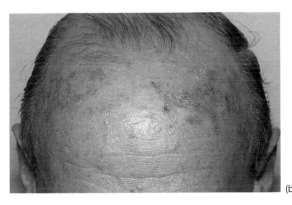
(b)

Fig. 18.7 Treatment of actinic keratoses with topical 5-fluorouracil. Actinic keratoses are common on the non-hair-bearing scalp skin of Caucasian males (a). Topical 5-fluorouracil cream was applied once a day for 3–4 weeks. After approximately 7 days the patient developed redness, scaling and soreness of the treated skin, particularly around existing keratoses (b). The treatment should be continued for the full course despite this reaction, which can be severe. Topical steroids can be used to reduce inflammation without reducing clinical effectiveness. This patient had a good result when assessed at 8 weeks, although there was one persistently thickened area which did not respond. Subsequent excision confirmed that this was a squamous cell carcinoma.

Solitary patches of Bowen's disease can be curetted, excised or treated by radiotherapy or cryotherapy.

The risks of all the destructive therapies described are site-dependent. All leave ulcers or erosions and since actinic keratoses and Bowen's disease commonly occur on the lower leg in elderly females with oedematous legs and poor peripheral circulation, there is risk of infection or delayed healing. By comparison, treated lesions on the head and neck heal rapidly.

5FU (Fig. 18.7) can be tried in the treatment of small superficial BCCs, although there are few large studies demonstrating its effectiveness. 5FU should not be used for the treatment of solid BCC. (Superficial BCC is a clinicopathological diagnosis. These tumours spread laterally rather deeply and are characteristically seen on the trunk.)

Further reading

Brodland DG & Zitelli JA (1992) Surgical margins for excision of primary cutaneous squamous cell carcinoma. *J Am Acad Dermatol* **27**: 241–248.

Emmett AJJ & Broadbent GG (1981) Basal cell carcinoma in Queensland. *Aust NZ J Surg* **51**: 576–590.

Emmett AJ & O'Rourke MGE (1991) (eds) *Malignant Skin Tumours* 2nd edn. Churchill Livingstone, Edinburgh.

Evans J & McCann BG (1990) A new protocol for the treatment of Stage 1 cutaneous malignant melanoma; interim results of the first 806 patients treated. *Br J Plast Surg* **43**: 426–430.

Lawrence CM (1993) Mohs surgery of basal cell carcinoma — a critical review. *Br J Plast Surg* **46**: 599–606.

Lawrence CM, Dahl MGC & Comaish JS (1986) Excision of skin malignancies without wound closure. *Br J Dermatol* **115**: 563–571.

Lawrence CM, Matthews JNS & Cox NH (1995) The effect of ketanserin on healing of fresh surgical wounds. *Br J Dermatol* **132**: 580–586.

Rowe DE, Carroll RJ & Day CL (1992) Prognostic factors for local recurrence, metastasis and survival rates in squamous cell carcinoma of the skin, ear and lip. *J Am Acad Dermatol* **26**: 976–990.

Zitelli JA (1983) Wound healing by secondary intention. *J Am Acad Dermatol* **9**: 407–415.

19: Management of complications

Immediate complications

Anxious patient

In local anaesthetic surgery the operator must gain the confidence of and establish a rapport with the patient. An anxious patient is better reassured with words and gentle handling than with sedative drugs. If necessary, oral temazepam given 1 hour before surgery can be used. Intravenous diazepam should be avoided because of the risk of respiratory depression and long recovery time. Background music may distract the patient, although personal earphones are usually impracticable because they obstruct the surgeon and hinder communication. Deaf patients should be encouraged to leave their hearing aids in whenever possible to facilitate conversation. Communication between staff should be confident and mutually supportive. Choose motivated and harmonious staff. The operation is not the time or place for a disagreement with a colleague.

Discourage outside interruptions. Patients lying on the table about to undergo a potentially painful operation feel very vulnerable and need to know that they have your full attention. Anxious patients are frequently reassured simply by being asked to hold a cotton swab over the injection site whilst waiting for the anaesthetic to take

effect and before cleaning the skin. Involve the patient in your conversation. Some patients will want to know what you are doing; others will not. Conversation about family, hobbies or a common interest will make the time pass faster and relax the patient. If patients start to panic, avoid manually restraining them but ensure they do not injure themselves. Stop the procedure temporarily if necessary, perhaps give the patient a drink and constantly reassure that all is well. Avoid getting frustrated with an anxious or frightened patient.

Remember that a forewarned patient is better prepared to accept reassurance so discuss potential immediate postoperative hazards such as bruising, swelling, loss of function, a black eye, periorbital oedema and tracking of blood to distant sites and at the end of the procedure warn again about avoiding alcohol, bending, stooping, exercise and aspirin (Table 19.1).

Intraoperative bleeding

Haemostasis is discussed in Chapter 5. If postoperative bleeding complications regularly occur, reassess your use of prophylactic pressure bandages and haemostasis techniques.

Haematoma formation

Bruising and swelling postoperatively are common, particularly when operating around the forehead or eyes. Bruising may track some distance from the wound site, e.g. to the jaw line from an operation on the upper lip, especially after extensive undermining. Coexisting aspirin or anticoagulant therapy and other factors (Table 19.2) may aggravate this. If a haematoma forms within hours of surgery, local pressure should be tried initially. Unfortunately, however, the local

Table 19.1 Standard advice for patients after surgery.

Go straight home
No strenuous exertion, bending or stooping
Rest with the feet up for 24 hours after surgery on the lower limb
Avoid alcohol (it encourages bleeding)
Use paracetamol rather than aspirin for pain relief
Apply continuous firm pressure for 20–30 minutes if bleeding occurs

Table 19.2 Haematoma risk factors.

Cause	Mechanism	Avoidance
Bleeding diathesis	Aspirin	Stop 7–10 days preoperatively
	Warfarin	Get INR < 2.5 if possible
	NSAID therapy	Stop 24–48 hours before
	von Willebrand's disease — history of prolonged bleeding after tooth extraction, etc.	Haematology referral
Poor technique	Inadequate perioperative haemostasis	Careful operating. Avoid over reliance on temporary adrenaline effect
	Retained dead space	Use subcutaneous sutures and pressure dressing to obliterate dead space
Site	Around eye	Warn patient about bending, stooping, strenuous exertion
	Lower limb	Use a support bandage
		Rest for 24 hours with legs up
	Arms and hand	Use an arm sling for first 24 hours

INR, international normalized ratio; NSAID, non-steroidal anti-inflammatory drug.

anaesthetic effect may have begun to wear off by this time and the patient may be unable to tolerate adequate pressure. If bleeding persists after 1–2 hours and the haematoma is still enlarging, the wound should be re-explored. The patient will need to be taken back to the operating room, more local anaesthetic injected and the bleeding point identified and diathermied or tied off, if a single bleeding vessel can be identified. The wound can then be resutured. If there is generalized ooze, as occurs in patients with a bleeding diathesis, a haemostatic dressing (Chapter 5) will have to be used. The wound can then be partially closed or allowed to heal by second intention (Fig. 19.1).

Cutting important structures

You should be familiar with the superficial anatomy of the area on which you plan to operate. In tumour surgery small cutaneous sensory nerves are commonly encountered and can be sacrificed without significant sensory loss, particularly on the central face (Fig. 8.7). Nerve ramifications at these sites are so multiple and small that the loss of a tiny branch will produce only localized temporary numbness. Injuries to motor nerves are potentially more catastrophic. Vulnerable

sites are listed in Chapter 8. An important nerve accidentally and knowingly divided during surgery is best resutured immediately to avoid painful neuroma formation and speed restoration of function. On the head and neck large arteries and veins can be tied off without causing major

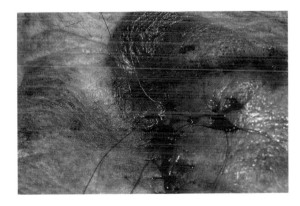

Fig. 19.1 Haematoma formation. This elderly woman had a large exophytic basal cell carcinoma on her cheek adjacent to her lower lid, which was excised and closed with an O-T repair. A haematoma formed and continued to enlarge, despite local pressure. Eventually the wound had to be re-explored and the bleeding sources diathermied. A haemostatic dressing was placed in the wound, which was partially resutured. Questioning revealed that she had taken aspirin a few days earlier.

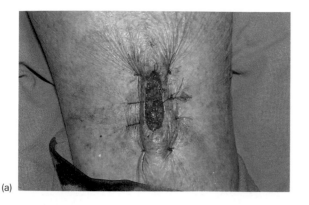
(a)

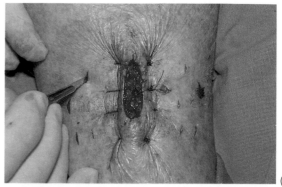
(b)

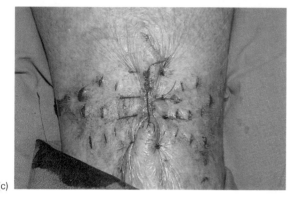
(c)

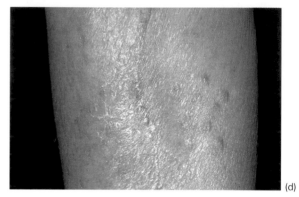
(d)

Fig. 19.2 Relaxing incisions. After excision of a superficial spreading melanoma on the leg, the oval-shaped defect (a) was closed but there was insufficient skin laxity to enable the edges to be apposed comfortably (b). Multiple relaxing incisions were made (c) and this made skin apposition possible. The dog ears (Fig. 13.6) were repaired and the wound closed. At suture removal 12 days later, the relaxing incisions had started to heal by second intention. The cosmetic effect was good at 4 months (d).

problems because there is such an excellent blood supply and collateral circulation at this site. Around the ear a deep incision may result in incision of the parotid gland. Saliva may be seen to flow from the cut surface and occasionally a salivary fistula may form. In both instances, if the parotid duct is patent, the problem can be solved by simple suturing of the fistula. If the lacrimal duct is severed it can be resutured by an expert, although this may only be possible at the time of surgery.

A difficult wound closure

If a defect proves to be difficult to close, a variety of techniques can be used to improve adjacent skin mobility (Table 19.3). Alternatively the wound can be allowed to heal by second intention (Chapter 18) or closed with a graft or flap. Skin mobility can be increased by undermining (Chapter 8), subcutaneous sutures or a surface pulley suture (Fig. 6.12b). In addition, relaxing incisions (Fig. 19.2), placed parallel to the incision and at the tensest part of the wound, allow the adjacent skin to be stretched. The resulting small diamond-shaped defects heal later by second intention. The technique is particularly useful for excisions on the lower leg. If there is a few hours' delay between excision and closure the adjacent skin can be stretched by drawing together the wound edges using a strong suture sited at some distance from the wound edge. Second-

Table 19.3 Methods for dealing with a difficult wound closure.

Increasing skin mobility
Undermining (Fig. 8.10)
Subcutaneous sutures (Fig. 6.11)
Pulley suture (Fig. 6.12b)
Relaxing incisions (Fig. 19.2)

Do not close the wound
Allow entire wound to granulate (Fig. 18.4)
Partial closure (Fig. 19.3)

Complex closure
Split- or full-thickness graft
Local flap

intention healing (Chapter 18) is a useful technique for some sites. This can also be employed with some of the techniques described above so that the wound is partially closed and a much smaller area is allowed to heal by second intention (Fig. 19.3). If the wound edges can only be apposed at the expense of producing extreme wound tension it is better to release some of the tension and allow the central portion of the wound to heal by second intention as the risk of wound infection is so great under these circumstances. Skin flaps, with or without tissue expansion, also produce excellent results. Skin grafts

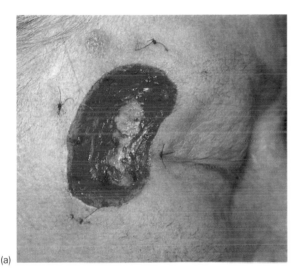

(a)

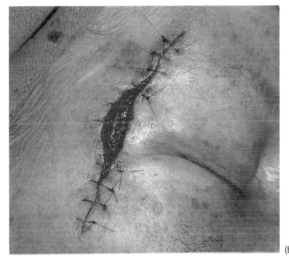

(b)

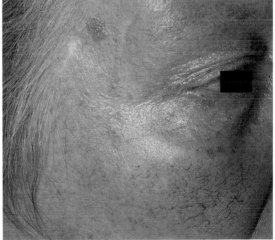

(c)

Fig. 19.3 Partial closure after basal cell carcinoma (BCC) excision. A large recurrent BCC has been excised using microscopically controlled excision. The defect (a) could only be partially closed without producing excessive tension and thereby placing the wound edges at risk from ischaemic necrosis and possibly distorting the lateral canthus of the eye. The central portion was therefore not sutured (b), but allowed to heal by second intention. The result (c) 6 months later was very good.

are technically easier to perform but may produce inferior cosmetic results. These techniques are beyond the scope of this book.

Delayed complications

Wound breakdown

Wound strength is less than 5% of the unwounded skin strength at the time of suture removal. Thus, immediately after suture removal the wound is vulnerable and may easily split open during sudden movement, particularly if the wound tension was excessive before suturing. The risk of dehiscence may be reduced by applying adhesive tape strips (Chapter 6) after suture removal. If wound tension is too great at the time of suturing this can be reduced by some of the methods listed in Table 19.3. The common methods used are adequate undermining (Chapter 8) and subcutaneous sutures (Chapter 6). Leaving surface sutures in for longer reduces the risk of wound breakdown but increases the risk of stitch marks remaining. Excessive tension at the time of closure will predispose to the risk of infection, which in turn impairs healing and increases the risk of dehiscence. If an uninfected wound bursts open it can be resutured. Alternatively it can be allowed to heal by second intention. If a wound becomes infected and then bursts, the infection must be treated and the wound allowed to heal by second intention.

Infection

Most wound infections are caused by *Staphylococcus aureus* and this organism usually originates from the subject's skin. This bacteria is more likely to be present if the skin surface is broken or crusted (Fig. 19.4). Approximately 5% of apparently healthy individuals carry this organism on their hand and arm skin and carriage increases to 15% in the axilla and 25% in the groin and perineum. Bacteria numbers can be reduced by the use of skin antiseptics but none will completely sterilize the skin (Chapter 2). If there is skin ischaemia caused by excessive skin-

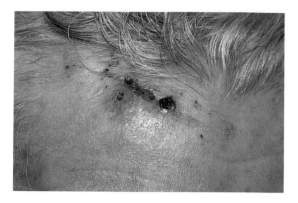

Fig. 19.4 Infected wound. A large abscess has formed under the suture line on this patient's wound. All the sutures should be removed and the pus drained. Topical and oral antibiotics are required. The wound should be allowed to heal by second intention.

edge or flap tension the presence of *S. aureus* will virtually guarantee a wound infection. Prophylactic oral and topical antibiotics may be used to prevent secondary infection, particularly if wound tension is considered to be less than optimal. When a wound becomes infected or an abscess develops (Fig. 19.4) in a sutured wound the sutures must be removed, the pus drained, bacteriological specimens taken and topical and systemic antibiotics started.

Incompletely excised tumours

A histology report that suggests a tumour has been incompletely excised must be viewed in the light of what was attempted. A diagnostic incisional biopsy, curettage or shave excision all inevitably result in histological specimens that show tumour present at the specimen margin (Chapter 21). When curettage has been correctly chosen and performed (Chapter 9) as the appropriate technique based on a sound preoperative diagnosis of the type of tumour, then no further treatment would be required apart from appropriate follow-up. Incisional or shave biopsy of a skin tumour would only have been done to aid diagnosis and hence plan further treatment. By contrast, if an attempt had been made to excise the tumour completely, further treatment may be required and this is discussed in Chapter 18.

Unexpected tumour

All excised lesions must be sent for histological examination. If an apparently benign lesion proves to be malignant the histology report must be interpreted in the light of what was done. If an attempt was made to excise, with a suitable margin of normal skin, a tumour that proves to be a basal cell carcinoma and the lesion was histologically completely excised, no further treatment is required. The patient should be followed up yearly for 5 years. Unlike squamous cell carcinoma, and with the exception of keratotic basal cell carcinomas, there is little risk of lymph node metastasis from basal cell carcinoma (Chapter 21). If malignancy was not suspected and no attempt was made to excise the lesion fully, or a shave or incisional biopsy was performed, the area should be re-excised. In the case of a basal or squamous cell carcinoma, this is best done using Mohs micrographic surgery to ensure complete removal (Fig. 18.3).

When the differential diagnosis of a skin nodule includes melanoma the lesion should always be excised down to fat with a 1–2 mm margin of normal skin, or the patient sent for an urgent specialist opinion (Chaper 18). If melanoma was considered in the differential diagnosis and the lesion fully excised the patient should be referred urgently for further surgery. It is wise to mention this possibility to the patient before initial excision. A similar excisional staging biopsy would normally be undertaken prior to definitive surgery (Table 18.5). By contrast, if a melanoma has been inadvertently curetted off or an incisional or shave biopsy performed, the patient's management may be adversely affected. There is a controversial but potential risk of early lymphatic spread following incisional biopsy of melanoma. Furthermore, since maximal tumour thickness must be known before appropriate surgical therapy is planned, incomplete histological examination of the original tumour should be avoided (Fig. 18.6). In these circumstances the diagnosis must be explained and the patient referred for further surgery (Chapter 18).

Sutures spitting

Vicryl and Dexon sutures may spit or be extruded through the skin. This presents as an area of granulation tissue along the suture line 2–4 weeks after closure (Fig. 6.2). The suture can be picked out or left to be expelled spontaneously and the area allowed to heal. Cosmesis is not usually affected, but any secondary infection caused by breach of the epidermis should be treated.

Delayed healing

Wound healing by second intention and after curettage and cryotherapy may be prolonged, especially on the lower limb. This must be distinguished from recurrence of the original lesion and self-induced or artefactual damage. Provided there is an adequate blood supply, any skin wound should heal normally provided it is kept clean, infection-free and any coexisting venous disease treated by compression bandaging. If the limb is ischaemic it is possible that the treatment site may be very difficult to heal. Therefore it is important to ensure that the patient has reasonable skin blood flow by assessing pulses, capillary flow and, if necessary, Doppler pressure measurements before embarking on destructive therapies on the lower limb. Remember that pyoderma gangrenosum may appear at skin injury sites and could be confused with delayed healing. Split-skin grafting of the delayed healing site can be done but at the expense of creating a donor site which may become the next delayed wound-healing site.

Eyelid oedema

Persistent lower-eyelid oedema following excisions on the lower eyelid is not uncommon and is due to division of lymphatics. This may take months to settle, but invariably does.

Late complications

Poor cosmesis (Table 19.4)

Before any surgical procedure discuss the possible cosmetic result with the patient and tell him/her that a scar will be created. Some patients have a misguided idea of what is possible and it is essential, particularly when something is removed for cosmetic reasons, that the patient understands that a scar is inevitable. It may be possible to reassure the patient that the final result will be an improvement on the current defect but if this is not the case, e.g. when excising a naevus on the back, let the patient know before surgery is done.

Patients with black or brown skin commonly develop hypo- or hyperpigmentation at skin injury sites, particularly after cryotherapy (Fig. 17.6). Plan the incision correctly (Chapter 13) so that it is aligned with the skin-crease or wrinkle lines (Fig. 8.1). Closure using the dog-ear repair technique (Chapter 13) may be preferable and produces a shorter scar than an equivalent elliptical excision.

Table 19.4 Risk factors for poor cosmetic results.

Risk factor	Hazard
Age	Risk of keloid and hypertrophic scar greatest in adolescence
Site	Keloid-prone sites: upper back, anterior central chest, upper arms, shoulders Stretched scar sites: limbs, upper back
Black skin	Risk of hypo- and hyperpigmented scars
Past history of thickened scars	Examine BCG site and any other scars
Cigarette smoker	Increased risk of ischaemic necrosis, particularly after complex repair
Unreal expectation	Patient may have an inaccurate idea of what can be achieved

BCG, Bacillus Calmette-Guérin.

Wound contracture

Wounds continue to contract after healing. This may present problems near the lower eyelid where contraction can precipitate ectropion formation in an individual with weak eyelid tone (Fig. 8.11).

Stitch marks

Stitch marks can be prevented by early removal of sutures, i.e. before 5 days. However, this is done at the risk of a burst wound. The use of tape strips and subcutaneous sutures will reduce the risk of wound dehiscence and thus allow surface sutures to be removed at an appropriate time. Monofilament suture materials (Chapter 6) produce less tissue reaction (Table 6.1) compared to silk and should be used in preference.

Keloid and hypertrophic scars

Keloids and hypertrophic scars are more common in young individuals, African-Caribbeans and at certain sites (Fig. 7.3). Hypertrophic or keloidal scars can be treated using the collagen-atrophying effect of corticosteroids. Intralesional steroids, 10–40 mg/ml triamcinolone, injected into the scar every 2–3 weeks four to six times may also help in hypertrophic scars (Fig. 19.5). Remember that triamcinolone injections may produce temporary hypopigmentation in black skin. Potent topical steroids, e.g. clobetasol propionate (Dermovate) or steroid tape, e.g. flurandrenolone (Haelan) tape, may be helpful. The tape carries less risk of steroid atrophy of the adjacent skin because only the scar is covered. Hypertrophic scars may improve with time but keloids persist. Silicone gel sheeting may help.

Stretched scars

Sutured wounds virtually never achieve the same strength as the unwounded adjacent skin. Even after 12 years the scar is only 40–80% as strong as the surrounding skin. A wound may look perfect when the sutures are removed but stretch several

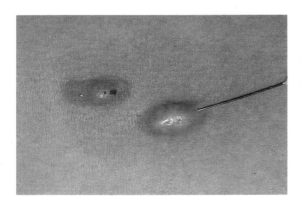

Fig. 19.5 Keloid injection of triamcinolone. Keloids can be injected with triamcinolone 10–40 mg/ml. This is painful and local anaesthetic injection may be required first. Because the keloid is so stiff and difficult to inject into, great pressure is required and this frequently results in the needle being forced off the syringe, resulting in the solution going everywhere. A Luer-lock glass syringe is thus helpful and a 30-gauge 0.5-in needle may make the injection less painful. Repeat injections are frequently required. Atrophy of the keloid collagen may occur but there is always the risk of steroid-induced atrophy in the surrounding normal skin.

weeks later, before the wound has reached its maximal strength. The risk of this happening is reduced by minimizing wound tension by correct wound-siting, adequate undermining and increasing wound strength using subcutaneous sutures and tape strips (Chapter 6). Patients should also be warned about the risks of strenuous activity that may stretch the area before the wound has had time to reach its maximal strength. Occasionally, despite all these efforts, scars particularly on the limbs and back of young or active individuals stretch. Wound correction can be attempted but requires great expertise.

Recurrent tumours

Recurrent basal cell carcinomas are more difficult to treat than primary tumours and are best dealt with by excision with histological margin control (Fig. 18.1).

Further reading

Bennett RG (1988) Keloid therapy. In: *Fundamentals of Cutaneous Surgery*. CV Mosby, St Louis.

Fewkes JL, Cheney ML & Pollack SV (1992) Complications. In: *Illustrated Atlas of Cutaneous Surgery*. JB Lippincott/Gower Medical, Philadelphia.

Harris DR (1979) Healing of the surgical wound. *J Am Acad Dermatol* 3: 197–207.

Mohs FE (1978) *Mohs Surgery*. Chemosurgery, microscopically controlled surgery for skin cancer. Charles C Thomas, Springfield.

Motley RJ & Holt PJA (1990) The use of meshed advancement flaps in the treatment of lesions on the lower leg. *J Dermatol Surg Oncol* 16: 346–348.

Salasche SJ (1986) Acute surgical complications: cause, prevention and treatment. *J Am Acad Dermatol* 15: 1163–1185.

Salasche SJ & Grabski WJ (1990) *Flaps for the Central Face*. Churchill Livingstone, New York.

Zachary C (1991) *Basic Dermatological Surgery*. Churchill Livingstone, New York.

20: Legal aspects of surgery in general practice

General practitioners who undertake surgical procedures may face a number of medico-legal problems if the result fails to meet the patient's expectations. These include complaints to the practice or the Health Authority (Health Board in Scotland and Northern Ireland), claims in negligence and, in extreme cases, referral to the General Medical Council. To minimize the risk, doctors should ensure that they have the requisite skill and knowledge to undertake the proposed procedure; that their facilities and equipment are adequate, and that care is taken to avoid the common causes of error. Preoperative counselling, including warning of potential risks, is imperative to ensure that a valid consent is obtained from the patient.

Complaints and discipline

New National Health Service (NHS) complaints procedures were introduced on the 1 April 1996. The aim being to provide a simple and fair system to resolve complaints speedily and wherever possible at a local level. All GP practices and NHS Trusts must have in place their own complaints procedures with the emphasis on accessibility, informality, speed and fairness to all concerned. Deciding what is not a complaint can itself be problematic. One suggested definition is 'an expression of dissatisfaction requiring a response'.

The golden rules for dealing with complaints in-house are; remain courteous, objective and professional throughout the procedure. Ensure that the facts are established before attempting to provide any response other than an acknowledgement. Maintain professional confidence at all times. The Terms of Service now require for a written record to be kept of all complaints but the written record should not be filed within the patient's record. Many complaints will be amenable to local resolution but if the complainant remains dissatisfied, he/she can ask for an independent review by the Health Authority. A non-executive director of the Authority termed 'the convenor' will consider the request.

Before deciding whether or not to convene a review panel, the convenor must obtain a statement signed by the complainant setting out his/her remaining grievances and why he/she is dissatisfied with the outcome of local resolution. The convenor and a lay chairperson of the regional review panel will then consider whether any further action short of establishing a panel can be taken to satisfy the complainant and whether establishing a panel would add further value to the process.

When the convenor is considering a clinical complaint, he/she must take appropriate clinical advice before reaching a decision but the final decision is for the convenor alone. Complainants denied an independent review have a right of 'appeal' to the ombudsman (Health Service Commissioner). The chairman of the independent review panel will have considerable discretion in deciding how best to investigate a particular case but it would be extremely unusual for there to be a formal hearing of both parties present. The panel will produce a report to be copied to the complainant, the practice and the Health Authority, reviewing the facts and where necessary making recommendations for further action. The report does not contain recommendations about disciplinary action. It would be for the Health Authority to decide whether or not any further action is necessary.

Although there will be no direct connection between the complaints procedure and disciplinary action, Health Authorities will be able to instigate a formal disciplinary investigation where this appears appropriate. In a disciplinary procedure, the Health Authority itself acts as complainant to a disciplinary panel appointed by another Health Authority. The function of the panel is to investigate the facts and decide whether or not there has been breach of the Terms of Service. The panel will then report back to the original (complaining) Health Authority who must then decide what action should be taken. Available sanctions will include a warning to comply more closely with the Terms of Service in future, a financial witholding and referral to the General Medical Council or NHS Tribunal.

There is no right of appeal for Health Authorities against the decision of a disciplinary panel, but the doctor will be able to appeal against a finding of a breach of the Terms of Service and against any penalty imposed by his/her own Health Authority. In England the appeal will be to the Family Health Services Special Health Authority; in Scotland, Wales and Northern Ireland to the Secretary of State.

Negligence

Doctors must ensure that they have adequate facilities to cope with the task in hand and any reasonably foreseeable complications. In the wake of acquired immunodeficiency syndrome (AIDS) and hepatitis, the British Medical Association has recommended that practices use autoclaves — not sterilizers. In view of this advice, it would be difficult to defend a practitioner against an allegation of negligence or a breach of the terms of service if a patient contracted an infection as a result of the use of sterilizers as opposed to autoclaves.

The courts require a doctor to keep abreast of current standards in respect of surgical procedures. Using an outdated surgical method with a higher incidence of complications will prove difficult to defend.

For a patient to succeed in a medical negligence action, the patient cum plaintiff must prove on the balance of probabilities that the doctor owed a duty of care to the patient (which is automatic where the doctor has embarked upon a therapeutic procedure); that the doctor breached that duty of care and that the patient suffered harm as a result of the breach of duty of care.

The standard of care in English law is referred to as the Bolam test, which requires doctors 'to act in accordance with a practice accepted as proper by a responsible body of medical men skilled in that particular art, even though a body of adverse opinion may also exist amongst medical men'. If a claim is to be defended successfully, the doctor will rely upon experts to testify that the care provided was of an appropriate standard. When undertaking surgical procedures, the general practitioner is not acting as a general practitioner but as a surgeon and so the appropriate experts will be surgeons with expertise in that particular field. It is no defence for a doctor to say 'I was only doing my best' or 'I did as well as the average general practitioner would have done in the circumstances'. To embark upon a procedure beyond your own level of skill is itself a breach of duty of care and invites a poor result.

The standards required under the terms of service and the Bolam test appear different. General practitioners arraigned before Medical Service Committees will be judged by their peers advising lay colleagues on the committee, whereas in the courts general practitioner surgeons must measure up to the standard required of specialists. The difference here may be more apparent than real in that, under both tests, the doctor must act within his/her own level of expertise, referring procedures that cannot be undertaken within the practice to others with the requisite facilities, experience and skill.

Lastly, the patient must prove that harm has been suffered which would not have occurred but for the negligence of the doctor.

Consent

Even when the result of the operation is as good as could be expected, a medical negligence claim may still succeed if the patient was given insufficient information to make an informed choice on whether or not to accept the procedure — or, to put it another way, if the consent was obtained negligently. For such a claim to succeed, patients have to prove that had they been warned of the risk which materialized, they would not have consented to the procedure.

For a consent to be valid, the patient must have the intellectual capacity to appreciate the implications of accepting or rejecting a particular treatment, be given sufficient information to enable a choice to be made and give the consent voluntarily.

English law requires the doctor to decide what information should be disclosed to the patient prior to canvassing consent. No hard-and-fast rule exists, but the factors to be considered include the seriousness of the potential complication, its frequency and the necessity of the proposed treatment. When a purely aesthetic procedure is contemplated, the duty to disclose potential risks is high; where a life-saving procedure is required, the duty is less severe but, in either case, if posed a direct question, the doctor must answer truthfully and as fully as the questioner requires.

A teenage girl attended her general practitioner complaining of a blemish over the sternal area. She asked if it could be removed and an excision was subsequently performed. No warning was given about possible scarring. Experts advise that a keloid scar was probable following an excision in the sternal area, even in Caucasian skin, and that to fail to warn of such scarring was indefensible.

Consent form (Fig. 20.1)

There is a commonly held belief that a consent form is in itself indisputable proof that valid consent was obtained. This is a triumph of myth over reality as consent forms are at best merely evidence that a valid consent was obtained. In the majority of cases, the validity of the consent will depend upon the adequacy of the counselling that took place prior to canvassing consent, the key points of which should be recorded in the patient's notes. Whilst consent forms may be useful for evidential purposes, there is no strict requirement to obtain written consent for procedures under local anaesthetic, although doing so

may be advisable where either the procedure or the patient is likely to prove difficult.

If an adult patient cannot understand the implications of giving or withholding consent to a procedure, that patient is in legal terms incompetent. This creates a dilemma, as in English law no one, not even the next of kin or the courts, can give valid consent to treatment on behalf of an incompetent adult. This problem was addressed by the House of Lords in the case of Re F. Their Lordships ruled that the fact that no consent could be obtained did not preclude treatment which in the view of a responsible body of medical opinion was in the best interests of the patient. Faced with an incompetent patient, doctors should provide whatever treatment is necessary to promote the best interests of their patient, notwithstanding the fact that no consent can be obtained.

Common sources of error

The majority of claims arising out of surgery in general practice result from:
- incomplete excision of a lesion;
- excessive scarring;
- severing a nerve or some other structure;
- postoperative infection and its sequelae;
- failure to obtain a histological diagnosis;
- failure to arrange the necessary follow-up.

Incomplete excision of a malignant lesion such as a squamous cell carcinoma results in the need for further surgical procedures to complete removal of the tumour. In one case, the failure to remove a squamous cell carcinoma from the pinna of the ear resulted in a second operation some months later, producing a poor cosmetic result. Experts advise that had the first excision been adequate, the need for a second operation and the removal of so much tissue would not have arisen. A settlement was achieved out of court.

A carpenter consulted his doctor about a lump in the upper arm. A clinical diagnosis of lipoma was made and the lump was excised. Histological diagnosis revealed that the lump was arising from the radial nerve. The patient lost the use of the extensor muscles below the elbow and received

CONSENT

Standard Consent Form

I, ... of... ,
            Name   *Address*

*hereby consent to undergo
 or
*hereby consent to...undergoing the
                                      Name of patient

operation/treatment of...
the nature and purpose of which have been explained to me by

Dr/Mr...

I also consent to such further or alternative operative measures or treatment
as may be found necessary during the course of the operation or treatment
and to the administration of general or other anaesthetics for any of these
purposes. No assurance has been given to me that the operation/treatment
will be performed or administered by any particular practitioner.

Signature .... Date ....
                *Patient/parent/guardian**

I confirm that I have explained the nature and purpose of this operation/
treatment to the person(s) who signed the above form of consent.

Signature .... Date ....
                Medical practitioner

* *Delete whichever is inapplicable.*

Fig. 20.1 Standard consent form.

substantial damages as he was no longer able to earn his living as a carpenter.

The General Medical Council

The General Medical Council may institute disciplinary proceedings when a doctor appears *seriously* to have disregarded or neglected professional duties towards a patient. The General Medical Council guidance includes the following:

You must take suitable and prompt action when necessary. This must include;
(a) an adequate assessment of the patient's condition, based on the history and clinical signs including, where necessary, an appropriate examination;
(b) providing or arranging investigations or treatment where necessary;
(c) referring the patient to another practitioner, when indicated.

In providing care you must:
(a) recognize the limits of your professional competence;
(b) be willing to consult colleagues;
(c) be competent when making diagnoses and when giving or arranging treatment;
(d) keep clear, accurate and contemporaneous patient records which report the

relevant clinical findings, the decisions made, information given to patients and any drugs or other treatment prescribed;
(e) keep colleagues well informed when sharing the care of patients;
(f) pay due regard to efficacy and the use of resources;
(g) prescribe only the treatment, drugs or appliances that serve patients' needs.

A question of serious professional misconduct may also arise from a complaint or information about the conduct of a doctor which suggests that the welfare of patients has been endangered by a doctor persisting in unsupervised practice of a branch of medicine without having the appropriate knowledge and skill or having acquired the experience which is necessary.

In its 1993 annual report, the General Medical Council reported a case in which a doctor had been found guilty of serious professional misconduct for disregarding professional responsibilities in relation to minor surgery. They reported the facts as follows:

The Professional Conduct Committee considered the case of a general practitioner who had been consulted by a patient complaining of pain in her left ear. The doctor discovered hard skin in the patient's ear and conducted minor surgery to remove this. However, the patient continued to suffer from discomfort and the doctor again excised pieces of skin on no less than three further occasions over the ensuing months. On each occasion he failed to send the excised material for biopsy and it was found by the PCC [Professional Conduct Committee] that he had therefore failed to place himself in a position in which he

could properly assess the patient's condition. It was also found that the doctor had delayed unduly before referring the patient for specialist investigation . . . furthermore he failed to make any record in the patient's notes concerning any of the treatment which he had provided.

The importance of notes

Should a general practitioner be accused of a breach of the terms of service, negligence or serious professional misconduct, the defence will rely heavily upon clinical records. Many defensible cases are lost because there are inadequate contemporaneous notes to rebut the allegations. Although doctors can say what they would normally have done in that situation, without clear written evidence to show what *actually* happened, the defence is inevitably compromised. Medical records are the cornerstone of a doctor's defence, and the test of their adequacy is whether or not the doctor can reconstruct the consultation from the medical records without relying on memory. This does not mean writing an essay on each and every consultation but recording the key points of the history and examination, including important negative findings. In the case of surgical procedures, warning about adverse outcomes should also be recorded, as should objective measurements such as the size of the lesion involved.

Further reading

(1993) *Consent and Confidentiality.* Medical Protection Society.
Pickersgill D (1992) *The Law and General Practice.* Radcliffe Medical Press, Oxford.

21: Histological interpretation

All specimens must be sent for histology, the only exception being tiny skin tags. Histological confirmation of the diagnosis is an essential part of the procedure; this confirms diagnostic accuracy and provides a safety net against important missed diagnoses. Moreover, if late complications arise, the histology report removes any doubts about the original diagnosis.

Handling specimens

Preservation

The specimen must be fixed in 10% formaldehyde solution. Alcohol is not an appropriate fixative as it causes significant artefact. Once in formaldehyde, specimens can be kept indefinitely at room temperature. Specimens could thus be sent at intervals to the laboratory, although this will delay the histology report. When several specimens are sent from one patient, they must all be placed in separate pots and labelled correctly so that they can be distinguished.

Orientation of specimen

If a biopsy needs to be orientated to identify the involved area or a critical margin, a suture can be placed at one pole of the specimen (Fig. 21.1) or one edge of the specimen painted with typists' correction fluid before fixation. The correction fluid should be allowed to dry before the specimen is dropped into the formaldehyde. This will adhere to the specimen throughout processing and on the final histology slide will appear as an opaque black line. The laboratory will orientate excisional biopsies completely differently from diagnostic incisional specimens.

Mounting

Curetted or fragile specimens are best mounted on to paper before fixation (Fig. 12.4). If left on the paper for 1–2 minutes before being dropped into the formaldehyde, they will adhere to the paper and the resulting conglomeration can be processed as a single piece rather than multiple free-floating fragments, many of which will be lost.

Specialized techniques

Immunofluorescence specimens

Normal skin taken from either the edge of the lesion or from a distant site is usually taken (Table 21.1). Specimens can be frozen in liquid nitrogen immediately. Alternatively the biopsy can be wrapped in gauze dampened with sterile normal saline, placed in a sterile container and stored for 24–48 hours at 4°C until processed.

Electron microscopy specimens

Only minute 2 mm^2 pieces of tissue are required. Specimens can be placed in formaldehyde or, better still, buffered glutaraldehyde.

Histology forms

Correct interpretation of the histological specimen depends critically on the clinical information given. The minimum information required are patient details, specimen site and nature and the differential diagnosis. If this cannot be given, the history and examination findings should be provided (Table 21.2).

Table 21.1 Specimens required for immunofluorescence.

Disease	Best type of skin to biopsy	Expected result
Bullous pemphigoid	Uninvolved perilesional skin	Linear IgG, C3 along the basement membrane zone
Pemphigus vulgaris	Uninvolved perilesional skin	Intercellular IgG and C3 between keratinocytes
Dermatitis herpetiformis	Uninvolved skin (usually buttock, because the scar will not show)	Granular IgA ± C3 at the top of dermal papillae
Discoid lupus erythematosus	Non-lesional and non-sun-exposed skin — systemic lupus erythematosus (SLE) Non-lesional and sun-exposed skin — SLE and subacute cutaneous LE Lesional and sun-exposed — discoid LE	Linear IgM, IgG, IgA and C3 along the basement membrane zone (lupus band test)

IgG, immunoglobulin G.

Table 21.2 Histology form details.

Referring doctor details	Name, practice address, telephone number
Patient details	Date of birth, sex, address
Urgent/routine	
Type of specimen	Skin, etc.
Site	e.g. right upper arm
Nature of biopsy	Curetted, excision, incisional or shave biopsy
Symptom	e.g. change in a mole
Duration	Increasing size 4 months
Examination findings	Pigmented papule 5 mm diameter
Differential diagnosis	Mole, ?blue naevus, exclude malignant change

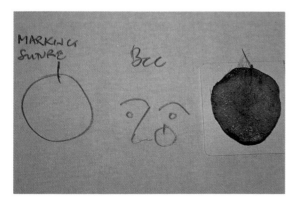

Fig. 21.1 Marking suture. The specimen can be very easily orientated by placing a suture at one point.

Laboratory handling of specimens

A skin biopsy has to pass through a range of steps before being ready to read as a haematoxylin and eosin-stained section (Table 21.3). When necessary, other stains or cell markers may be requested by the pathologist. The fastest practical time taken to process the specimen is 24 hours, although 48 hours is more realistic. When the specimen is received, the pathologist examines and describes the specimen, and on the basis of the information provided and the nature of the specimen, decides how the biopsy should be trimmed before being processed. Trimming involves cutting the biopsy into pieces so that sections will be taken from the appropriate parts of the biopsy — although the word suggests it, no tissue is discarded! For excisional biopsies a transverse section through the narrowest margin

Table 21.3 Stages in the preparation of a skin slide.

Specimen received in formaldehyde, details checked
Specimen examined, described and trimmed
Fixation in 10% formaldehyde for 24 hours
Specimen processed in paraffin wax
Sections cut
Sections stained
Coverslip applied
Slide ready to read

and cruciate sections at 90° to this are usually taken (Fig. 21.2). Incisional biopsies from inflammatory skin disease and small tumours or suspect melanomas are processed by taking transverse sections through the block. In a suspect melanoma these will be taken across the width of the elliptical biopsy, whereas longitudinal sections may be taken for inflammatory skin disease so that the maximum length of skin is examined on one slide. After being fixed and embedded in paraffin, the various pieces created by trimming the biopsy are stained, mounted and examined histologically.

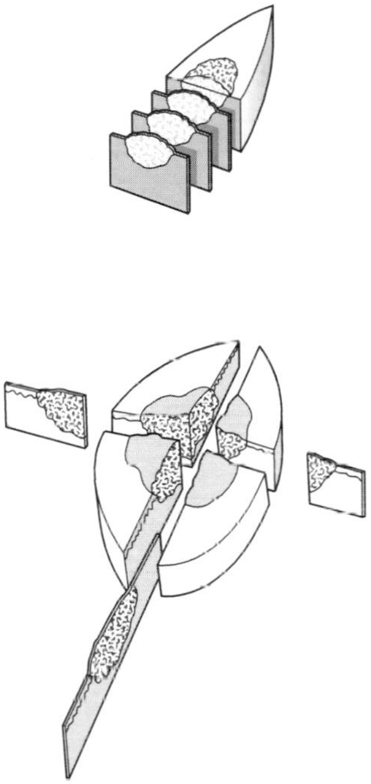

Interpretation of slides

The histological appearances of inflammatory skin diseases are rarely specific and the pathologist's ability to interpret the histology depends to a large extent on the clinical information and differential diagnosis provided. In some situations it is necessary to fit the clinical and histological features together to arrive at the diagnosis. There are relatively few inflammatory skin diseases with specific histological changes, so that whilst the pathological process (eczema, infection, etc.) can be described, the cause will not be apparent.

Histological terms

A variety of terms are used to describe skin histological appearances. These sometimes give rise to confusion. A few of the common ones are explained here.

(a)

(b)

Fig. 21.2 Sectioning skin specimens. Biopsies of suspected melanomas are trimmed so that multiple vertical sections are taken transversely through the specimen (bread-loaf technique; a). In inflammatory dermatoses the sections may be taken through the length of the specimen so that as much as possible of the specimen is examined on one slide. Skin tumours are commonly sectioned centrally across the potentially narrowest margin and cruciate sections taken at right angles to these; thus, only a small portion of the specimen cut edge is examined and tumour may extend beyond the excision margin, despite apparently being fully excised (b).

Histological term	Explanation
Acanthosis	Thickening of the epidermis
Acantholysis	Epidermal keratinocytes are connected by desmosomes. These are visible using a light microscope as tiny prickles on the cell border running from cell to cell, hence the term prickle (syn. spinous) cell for this epidermal layer. When these connections are damaged or poorly formed, the unattached, prickle-free or acantholytic cells float free within the epidermis. Acantholytic cells are seen in blistering diseases and malignant acantholysis occurs in epidermal cancers, e.g.

	Bowen's disease and squamous cell carcinoma.		between the granular layer of the epidermis and the deepest malignant melanocyte (Chapter 18)
Basal cell carcinoma (BCC)	Several BCC histological growth patterns are recognized, including adenoid, solid (Fig. 21.3), cystic, mixed, morphoeic, etc. Histological types likely to recur more frequently include morphoeic and infiltrative-pattern BCC. Basi-squamous or keratotic BCCs have metastatic potential and should be treated as squamous cell carcinomas	Dyskeratosis	Faulty keratinization producing prematurely keratinized cells. Seen in malignant (Bowen's disease) and benign (Darier's disease) conditions
		Dysplasia	Cellular change in the epidermis with early neoplastic features. The keratinocytes vary in size with loss of the normal orderly reduction in size in the higher levels of the epidermis
Basal cell papilloma	Another term for a seborrhoeic wart		
Benign squamous papilloma	Can be either a viral wart, seborrhoeic keratosis or other benign keratinocyte lesion.	Hypergranulosis	Thickening of the granular layer of the epidermis
		Hyperkeratosis	Thickening of the stratum corneum
Compound naevus	A mole showing nests or groups of naevus cells in both the dermis and junction between the dermis and epidermis	Intradermal naevus	A mole showing nests or groups of naevus cells in the dermis only
Clark's level	A method of estimating tumour invasion in malignant melanoma. Clark's level I = melanoma-*in-situ;* level II = melanoma extends into papillary dermis only; level III = extends up to but not into the reticular dermis; level IV = extends into the reticular dermis; level V = extends into subcutaneous fat. Usually this is less important than the depth of tumour infiltration, measured in millimetres (Breslow thickness)	Intraepidermal squamous cell carcinoma	Bowen's disease. Squamous cell carcinoma within the epidermis that has not yet broken through the basement membrane zone
		Junctional naevus	A mole showing nests or groups of naevus cells in the junction between the dermis and epidermis only
		Lentigo	Pigment cells extend continuously along the basal layer of the epidermis. Lentigo simplex does not progress to lentigo maligna.
Depth of invasion	Survival after melanoma excision relates to tumour thickness. This is measured in millimetres as the distance	Lentigo maligna	As above, except that the melanocytes are malignant. Between 10 and 20% of lentigo maligna go on to develop into lentigo maligna melanoma

Lentigo maligna melanoma	A melanoma arising in a lentigo maligna. The prognosis depends on tumour depth, as with all melanomas
Liquefaction (hydropic) degeneration	Damage to the basal layer of the epidermis, producing vacuoles and ultimately death of the basal cells. This is seen in lichen planus, some drug eruptions and discoid lupus erythematosus
Melanoma-in-situ	Malignant melanocytes within the epidermis but not breaching the basement membrane zone.
Microabscess	A small collection of inflammatory cells in the epidermis or just beneath the epidermis within the epidermis. There are three types:

Microabscess type	Cell type	Disease
Munro	Neutrophils	Psoriasis
Pautrier	Lymphocytes	Mycosis fungoides
Papillary	Neutrophils	Dermatitis herpetiformis
	Eosinophils	Bullous pemphigoid

Naevus	Histologically used to describe mole cells (melanocytic cells). Used clinically to describe pigment naevi and other birthmarks such as naevus sebaceous, naevus flammeus, strawberry naevus, etc.
Pagetoid	Spread of foreign cancer cells within the epidermis similar in pattern to that seen in breast skin affected by Paget's disease (intraduct carcinoma of the breast). Pagetoid spread occurs in Paget's disease, mycosis fungoides and extramammary Paget's disease

Parakeratosis	Retention of keratinocyte nuclear remnants in the stratum corneum. A feature of psoriasis and conditions in which keratinocyte differentation is abnormal
Spongiosis	Oedema between epidermal keratinocytes. An important feature of acute or subacute eczema

Expected results

Excised skin tumours must always be sent for histology to confirm the diagnosis and to demonstrate, as far as possible, that the tumour was completely excised (Fig. 21.3). Complete excision can only be considered probable if histologically the specimen appears to show that the tumour was fully removed and an attempt was made to excise the tumour. Note that this only refers to the sections that have been examined and does not guarantee adequate removal in routine histology processing techniques. If an incisional or shave biopsy was done and yet the report suggests that the tumour was fully excised, it must be assumed that the histology report is spurious and the tumour has been incompletely excised (Chapter 18).

A biopsy obtained after curettage (Fig. 21.4) or shave (Fig. 21.5) excision of a skin tumour will, by its very nature, always result in a specimen that potentially shows tumour extending to the edge. It should be remembered that curette reports only provide histological confirmation of the tumour and no information on adequacy or otherwise of treatment (Chapter 9).

Unexpected histology results

Unexpected histology results may need to be confirmed by the laboratory. If the suggested diagnosis is not compatible with the clinical appearance or differential diagnosis the histology should be reviewed, if possible by the physician and pathologist together, to ensure that a mistake has not

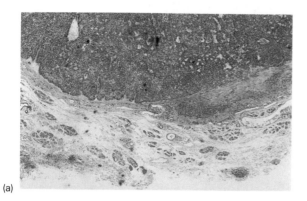
(a)

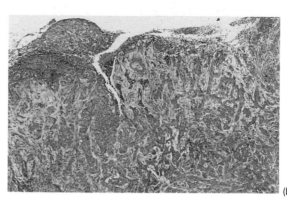
(b)

Fig. 21.3 Basal cell carcinoma (BCC) tumour margins. Some tumours have a well-defined border with a typical palisaded edge. A margin of normal skin around this is very suggestive of complete excision (a). Other BCCs have a more aggressive growth pattern with multiple tongues of tumour spreading out at irregular margins. This type of tumour may spread beyond the visible boundary and histological evidence of complete tumour removal is not always certain (b).

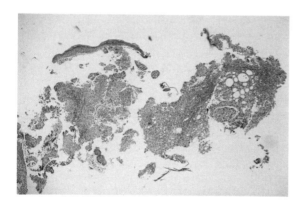

Fig. 21.4 Curettage specimen of basal cell carcinoma. Curetted specimens contain only fragments taken from the centre of the tumour. The margins always contain tumour. Curettage specimens provide no information about adequacy of treatment.

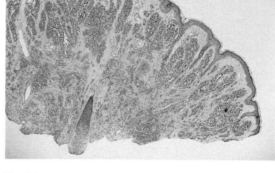

Fig. 21.5 Shave excision specimen. A shave excision of a simple benign compound naevus shows clumps of naevus cells present up to the base of the lesion as the incision has been taken through the mole. Persistent hairs and pigmentation occur in approximately a third of patients.

been made. Regular meetings between the pathologist and clinician to review selected specimens are very helpful in fostering an understanding of each other's needs and expectations.

Further reading

Lever WF & Schaumburg-Lever G (1989) *Histopathology of the Skin*, 7th edn. JB Lippincott, Philadelphia.

Appendix: manufacturers' details

Chapter 2: Equipment

Instrument suppliers and manufacturers

Albert Waeschle, Surgical Dental and Laboratory Supplies, 123/5 Old Christchurch Road, Bournemouth BH1 1EX.

Aesculap Ltd (formerly Downs Surgical), Parkway Close, Parkway Industrial Estate, Sheffield S3 4WJ. Tel: 01742 730346

DePuy Health Care, (formerly Thackray's), Millshaw House, Manor Hill Lane, Leeds LS11 8LQ. Tel: 01532 706000

Rockett's of London, Imperial Way, Watford, Herts WD2 4XX. Tel: 01923 39791

Compartmented trays

Rockett's, (see above)

Medical Plastics Division, 18 Longfield Road, Sydenham, Lemington Spa, Warwick

Chapter 3: Sterilization of surgical equipment

Smiths Industries Medical Systems, (manufacture autoclaves), Eschmann Equipment, Peter Road, Lancing, West Sussex BN15 8TJ. Tel: 01903 753322

Chapter 4: Local anaesthetics

Fine needles

30-gauge 0.5-in long (0.3 × 13 metric)

Microlance Becton Dickinson, UK Ltd
Between Towns Road, Cowley, Oxford OX4 3LY. Tel: 01865 748844

27-gauge 1.5-in long (0.4 × 40 metric)

Sterican B Braun Medical Ltd, Braun House, 13–14 Farnbourgh Close, Illsbury Vale Industrial Park, Stock Lane, Illsbury

Chapter 6: Suture materials and knot tying

Sterile skin-closure strips

Steristrips 3M

Leukostrip, Bejersdorf UK Ltd, Yeoman's Drive, Blakelands, Milton Keynes, Bucks MK14 5LS.

Chapter 7: Preoperative assessment and preparation

Template bleeding time estimations

Simplate-II, Organon Teknika Corp, Durham, North Carolina USA

Chapter 9: Curettage

Spoon Curette

Various-sized (3–6 mm), e.g. Lang Steel double-ended scoop (Downs catalogue number HM 135-05-F)

Ring curette

Disposable ring curettes:
Stiefel UK
Fox curette (3–6 mm) (Albert Waeschle catalogue number 28-188-01)

Chapter 11: Cautery and electrodesiccation

Cautery machines

Aesculap (Downs) catalogue

Cautery tips

Aesculap (Downs) catalogue. Cautery burners extra small 'for eye work' pattern no. 3

Chapter 15: Nail avulsion and ingrown toenail

Bailey Instrument Ltd, (chiropody set), Khyber House, 12 Chatham Road, Old Trafford, Manchester M16 0DR. Tel: 0161 860 5849

Chapter 17: Cryotherapy

Cryotherapy equipment

Cryac spray. Practice Management Systems Ltd, The Clockhouse, 145B Hughenden Road, High Wycombe, Bucks HP13 5PN. Tel: 01494 474811
CryoJet spray. Cryogenic Technology Ltd, Unit 2, Goods Road, Belper, Derbyshire DE5 1UU. Tel: 01773 821515

Histogreeze. Utermohlen Medical Care, UK distributors: Thames Laboratories, Abbey Road, The Industrial Estate, Wrexham, Cllwyd LL13 PW. Tel: 01978 661351

Liquid nitrogen supplies

British Oxygen, Sales Division, 10 Priestley Road, Guildford, Surrey GU2 5XY. Tel: 01483 579857
Cryoservice Ltd, Blackpole Trading Estate, Blackpole Road, Worcester WR3 8SG. Tel: 01905 754500

Chapter 19: Management of complications

Absorbable haemostatic dressings

Surgicel. Absorbable haemostat. Johnson & Johnson. Suitable size for dermatological surgery is 1.2×5 cm. Sterilized in double-wrapped sachets
Kaltostat. Calcium/sodium alginate fibre dressing. BritCair Ltd. Smallest size is 15×20 cm

Silicone gel sheeting

Cica-Care (Smith & Nephew), Silastic gel (Dow-Corning), Silgel, (Nagosil, PO Box 21, Douglas, Isle of Man)

Index

Page numbers in *italics* refer to figures, those in **bold** refer to tables. Word-by-word arrangement of entries is used.